CHAIR YOGA F(SENIORS

Revitalize Your Golden Years with Chair Yoga Through A Collection of Gentle Exercises For Balance, Posture Mobility and Strength

Mia Wellspring

Table of Contents

Introduction

Chair yoga is a gentle and accessible form of yoga specially designed for seniors and individuals with limited mobility. It offers all the benefits of traditional yoga, such as improved flexibility, balance, and relaxation, but it can be practiced while seated in a chair or using the chair for support.

This form of yoga is particularly well-suited for seniors because it helps maintain and improve physical and mental well-being without requiring them to get down on the floor or engage in strenuous poses. Chair yoga incorporates gentle stretches, breathing exercises, and relaxation techniques that promote better posture, joint health, and reduced stress.

The beauty of chair yoga is that it can be adapted to various fitness levels and physical abilities, making it an inclusive practice for everyone. Chair yoga might be modified to match your unique requirements and preferences, regardless of the fact that you are just starting out with yoga or are an experienced practitioner. Plus, it can easily be practiced in the comfort of your own home or as part of a group class at a local community center or senior center.

As we explore chair yoga in more depth, you'll discover its many benefits and learn how to get started on a journey towards improved physical and mental well-being. So, if you're a senior looking to enhance your overall health, flexibility, and inner calm, chair yoga might be the perfect practice for you.

Importance of Physical and Mental Well-being for Seniors

Physical and mental well-being are of paramount importance for seniors as they enter the golden years of their lives. This crucial phase of life, often characterized by retirement and increased leisure time, can be immensely rewarding when accompanied by good health and a sound state of mind. The significance of physical & mental well-being in the lives of seniors cannot be overstated, as it not only enhances the quality of their daily existence but also plays a pivotal role in extending their life expectancy and ensuring a fulfilling, independent, and dignified aging process.

Maintaining physical well-being is a cornerstone of healthy aging. As individuals grow older, their bodies undergo a series of changes that can impact their overall health and mobility. Regular physical activity, a balanced diet, and preventive healthcare measures are essential components of promoting physical well-being among seniors. Engaging in activities that encompass strength training, cardiovascular exercises, and flexibility routines can help seniors maintain muscle mass, bone density, and joint flexibility. This, in turn, reduces the risk of falls and fractures, which can have severe consequences for older individuals. A nourishing diet abundant in essential vitamins, minerals, and dietary fiber aids immune system functionality and reduces the likelihood of enduring chronic ailments like heart disease, diabetes, and osteoporosis. By actively participating in their healthcare and adhering to preventive measures, seniors can not only increase their longevity but also enhance their overall quality of life.

Equally critical to the well-being of seniors is their mental health. The aging process often comes with its unique set of challenges, such as coping with loss, adjusting to retirement, and dealing with the physical limitations that can accompany aging. Consequently, maintaining mental well-being is essential to navigate these challenges successfully. Social engagement and emotional support are vital components of mental well-being among seniors. Keeping a busy social life, being involved in activities in the community, and tending to one's relationships with one's family and friends are all important aspects of a healthy lifestyle which can provide seniors with a strong support network that helps combat loneliness and depression. Additionally, seniors can benefit from activities that stimulate cognitive function, such as puzzles, reading, or learning new skills. These activities not only keep the mind sharp but also provide a sense of purpose and accomplishment.

Furthermore, it is crucial to recognize the intricate connection between physical and mental well-being in seniors. Physical health issues can have a profound impact on mental health, and vice versa. Chronic pain, for instance, it has the potential to result in depression and isolation from social interactions. Similarly, depression can play a role in diminishing the drive to engage in physical activities and take care of oneself. By addressing both aspects of well-being simultaneously, seniors can achieve a more holistic and balanced approach to aging.

Benefits of Chair Yoga for Seniors

What are the advantages of engaging in chair yoga? Modified chair yoga postures engage many of the same muscle groups as traditional yoga poses, yielding comparable health benefits. Chair yoga practice can:

1. Enhance balance and flexibility: Maintaining balance and flexibility is crucial for overall health and independence, reducing the risk of injury as individuals age. A study conducted in 2010 among older adults in a retirement community who practiced chair yoga twice a week for 12 weeks revealed significant improvements in lower-body flexibility and static balance. This led to reduced fear of falling and increased confidence in their physical capabilities.

2. Improve muscle tone and strength: While traditional yoga is known to enhance strength across all age groups, a 2021 review indicates that chair yoga can help older adults develop and sustain muscle strength. Chair-based exercises were found to enhance upper and lower body function, a particularly important benefit as muscle mass tends to decline with age, potentially resulting in reduced strength and function.

3. Elevate mood and mental well-being: The practice of yoga has been associated with mental health benefits, including reduced anxiety and improved mood, a phenomenon that extends to various yoga styles, including chair yoga. In a small-scale study involving older adults who attended chair yoga classes once a week, participants reported notable improvements after three months, including decreased stress, improved mood, and fewer panic attacks. They also experienced an overall enhancement in their health, physical function, and social well-being.

4. Assist in managing chronic conditions: Chair yoga, when performed while seated, may be beneficial in helping individuals manage chronic health conditions like Type 2 diabetes. A pilot study observed the effects of a 10-min chair yoga program on people with diabetes who received standard care and were encouraged to incorporate the routine into their daily lives. Participants demonstrated enhancements in their blood sugar levels, heart rate, and blood pressure.

5. Alleviate chronic pain: Approximately 20% of adults contend with chronic pain that can significantly disrupt their daily lives. Emerging research suggests that yoga may serve as an effective alternative for managing chronic pain. One study found that practicing chair yoga could potentially help older adults reduce pain and combat fatigue associated with conditions like osteoarthritis.

How to Use This Book

This book serves as a comprehensive guide to chair yoga tailored for older adults. It emphasizes the importance of physical & mental well-being for seniors and the benefits of chair yoga. The book covers the history, philosophy, and safety guidelines of chair yoga. It offers practical sections with detailed explanations of chair yoga poses, breathing techniques, and relaxation exercises, all adapted to seniors' needs. Readers are encouraged to integrate chair yoga into their daily routines, adapting practices to their abilities and needs. The book emphasizes celebrating progress, maintaining consistency, and addressing common concerns through FAQs and troubleshooting. Ultimately, it acts as a trusted companion on the journey to enhanced well-being in senior years.

Disclaimer: Remember, your safety is paramount. Prior to beginning any fresh exercise routine, it is essential to discuss the matter with a qualified medical professional beforehand. By engaging in the exercises or activities mentioned, you acknowledge and agree that you are doing so at your own risk

Chapter 1:

Understanding Chair Yoga

What is Chair Yoga?

Chair yoga is a uniquely adaptable and gentle form of yoga that offers a diverse range of postures and exercises, all designed to be performed while seated or with the assistance of a chair. It has emerged as a highly inclusive and accessible practice, catering to individuals with physical disabilities, seniors looking for a more accommodating approach to yoga, beginners seeking a gradual introduction to yoga, and even seasoned practitioners aiming to fine-tune specific aspects of their practice.

For those with physical disabilities or elderly individuals who might find traditional yoga sessions physically demanding, chair yoga provides an excellent alternative. It accommodates a wide spectrum of physical abilities, making it a welcoming and comfortable space for people who may have otherwise felt excluded from the world of yoga. In chair yoga classes, participants can expect to engage in a variety of movements, stretches, and poses that harness the supportive framework of a chair, allowing them to experience the myriad benefits of yoga without the need to get down onto the floor.

Additionally, chair yoga serves as an invaluable tool within the broader yoga community. In standard Hatha yoga classes, instructors often incorporate elements of chair yoga to provide support and accessibility for participants who struggle with balance or encounter difficulties when transitioning to and from the floor. These chair-based modifications enable a more inclusive environment within yoga studios, ensuring that everyone, regardless of their physical condition or level of experience, can fully engage in the practice.

Chair yoga is not just about accessibility; it also offers a gentle yet effective approach to yoga that emphasizes mindfulness, breath control, and gradual progression. It allows individuals to delve into the essence of yoga, focusing on the mind-body connection and the meditative aspects of the practice. This more gentle style of yoga can be exceptionally advantageous for those in search of stress reduction, enhanced mental clarity, and an elevated sense of overall well-being. It offers a supportive atmosphere for self-exploration and individual development.

History and Origins of Chair Yoga

Chair yoga is a distinct and accessible form of yoga practice where individuals perform yoga postures while seated on a chair or utilize a chair for support while standing. This yoga approach boasts a deep-rooted history, originating in ancient India, which establishes it as one of the earliest documented forms of yoga.

The origins of chair yoga can be linked to the ancient Indian tradition of yoga, which dates back more than 5,000 years. In its classical manifestation, yoga encompasses a diverse array of physical, mental, and spiritual practices with the goal of attaining equilibrium, harmony, and overall well-being. Over millennia, as yoga evolved and diversified, it adapted to cater to the unique needs and abilities of different individuals.

Chair yoga, as it is known today, is the result of this evolutionary process. It was developed to make the profound benefits of yoga accessible to a broader audience, particularly those who may have physical limitations, mobility challenges, or difficulty with traditional floor-based yoga postures.

The advantages of chair yoga are numerous and wide-ranging. This practice offers an array of physical benefits, including enhanced flexibility through gentle stretches and movements. It promotes better circulation, helping to oxygenate the body and rejuvenate tired muscles. Moreover, chair yoga can provide relief from common discomforts, such as back pain, by engaging the core muscles and improving posture.

Beyond the physical advantages, chair yoga is highly regarded for its ability to reduce stress and promote relaxation. Through controlled breathing techniques and mindfulness exercises, practitioners can experience a sense of calm and mental clarity. This can be particularly beneficial in our fast-paced, stress-inducing modern lives.

Principles and Philosophy of Chair Yoga

The principles and philosophy of chair yoga are grounded in the broader philosophy of yoga itself, emphasizing unity, mindfulness, and holistic well-being. However, chair yoga introduces unique considerations and adaptations to make the practice accessible to individuals who may have limited mobility or physical challenges. Here are the key principles and philosophical underpinnings of chair yoga:

1. **Inclusivity and Accessibility**: Chair yoga embodies the principle of inclusivity, aiming to make the benefits of yoga available to a diverse range of individuals, regardless of age,

ability, or physical condition. It acknowledges that yoga is not limited to those who can perform complex postures on the mat but can be adapted to suit the needs of everyone.

2. **Adaptation and Modification**: The philosophy of chair yoga emphasizes the adaptability and modification of traditional yoga poses to accommodate participants' unique physical circumstances. This principle underscores that yoga is not a rigid set of postures but a flexible practice that can be tailored to the individual.

3. **Mind-Body Connection**: Chair yoga encourages participants to cultivate a strong mind-body connection. By focusing on the breath, sensations, and movements during the practice, individuals develop greater awareness and presence. This principle aligns with the core philosophy of yoga, which seeks to unite the body and mind.

4. **Acceptance and Non-Judgment**: Chair yoga fosters an environment of self-acceptance and non-judgment. Participants are encouraged to work within their own capabilities, recognizing that each person's journey is unique. This principle aligns with the yogic concept of "ahimsa" or non-violence, which extends to self-compassion.

5. **Balancing Effort and Ease**: The philosophy of chair yoga emphasizes finding the balance between effort and ease. Participants are guided to exert effort in a posture or movement while respecting their body's limits. This principle reflects the yogic principle of "sthira sukham asanam," which translates to finding steadiness and comfort in a pose.

6. **Breath Awareness and Pranayama**: Breath awareness is central to chair yoga. Practitioners are guided to synchronize their breath with movements, promoting relaxation, and reducing stress. The practice of pranayama (breath control) is often integrated, offering participants tools to manage their energy and emotions.

7. **Mindfulness and Meditation**: Chair yoga incorporates mindfulness practices and meditation techniques. These aspects encourage participants to cultivate present-moment awareness, promoting mental clarity and inner peace. This aligns with the broader yogic philosophy of self-awareness and self-realization.

8. **Holistic Well-being**: The philosophy of chair yoga recognizes that well-being extends beyond the physical body. It addresses mental, emotional, and spiritual aspects, aiming to create a holistic sense of wellness. This principle resonates with the ancient yogic understanding of the interconnectedness of all aspects of life.

9. **Personal Empowerment**: Chair yoga promotes personal empowerment by offering participants tools to enhance their physical and mental well-being. This principle aligns with the broader yogic philosophy of self-mastery and self-empowerment.

Safety Guidelines and Precautions

Safety guidelines and precautions are essential when practicing chair yoga, especially for individuals who may have physical limitations or health concerns. Ensuring a safe and comfortable practice is paramount. Here are some key safety guidelines and precautions to keep in mind:

1. **Consult with a Healthcare Professional**: Prior to commencing any fresh exercise regimen, such as chair yoga, it's prudent to seek advice from a healthcare professional, particularly if you have preexisting health conditions or specific concerns. They can provide guidance on whether chair yoga is suitable for you and offer specific recommendations.

2. **Choose the Right Chair**: Select a stable and sturdy chair with a flat seat and a straight back. Avoid chairs with wheels, rocking chairs, or chairs with arms that hinder movement. The chair should provide adequate support for your back and legs.

3. **Wear Comfortable Clothing**: Dress in loose-fitting, comfortable clothing that allows for ease of movement. Footwear is generally not needed for chair yoga, but non-slip socks can provide extra grip if desired.

4. **Set Up in a Safe Space**: Ensure you have enough space around the chair to move your arms and legs freely without obstacles. Clear the area of any potential tripping hazards.

5. **Practice Mindful Awareness**: Pay close attention to your body and its sensations throughout the practice. Listen to your body's signals and respect its limits. If you experience any pain or discomfort, stop the movement immediately.

6. **Use Props and Modifications**: Chair yoga often involves the use of props like cushions, blocks, or resistance bands to enhance comfort and support. Utilize these props as needed to adapt poses to your needs.

7. **Warm-Up and Cool Down**: Initiate your chair yoga session with mild warm-up exercises to ready your body for motion. Likewise, end with a cool-down to gradually return your body to a resting state.

8. **Proper Alignment**: Pay close attention to proper alignment in each pose. Your instructor (if you're in a class) or a knowledgeable resource should guide you in achieving correct alignment to prevent strain or injury.

9. **Avoid Overstretching**: Be cautious not to overstretch your muscles or joints. Stretch to a point where you feel a gentle pull but not to the point of pain. Remember that chair yoga is about gradual progress.

10. **Breathe Mindfully**: Focus on controlled and mindful breathing throughout your practice. Avoid holding your breath, which can create tension.

11. **Stay Hydrated**: Keep yourself hydrated by drinking water both prior to and following your workout, especially if your chair yoga session is longer or you are working up a sweat.

Do's and Don'ts for Seniors

Dos and don'ts are essential to consider when seniors engage in chair yoga or any other form of exercise. Ensuring a safe and enjoyable experience is crucial for promoting their well-being. Here are some dos and don'ts specifically tailored for seniors practicing chair yoga:

Dos:

1. **Consult Your Doctor**: Do consult your healthcare provider before starting any new exercise regimen, including chair yoga. Your doctor can offer insights into any specific precautions or modifications you should follow based on your medical history.

2. **Choose a Suitable Chair**: Do select a stable and sturdy chair with a straight back and flat seat. The chair should provide proper support for your posture during the practice.

3. **Listen to Your Body**: Do pay close attention to your body's signals. Practice mindfulness and only move within your comfort zone. If a movement feels uncomfortable or painful, stop immediately.

4. **Warm-Up and Cool Down**: Do begin your session of chair yoga with some light warm-up exercises so that your body is ready for the activity that will follow. Likewise, end with a cool-down to gradually relax your muscles and bring your heart rate back to normal.

5. **Use Props**: Do use props like cushions, blocks, or resistance bands as needed. Props can enhance comfort and support, allowing you to safely explore various poses.

6. **Focus on Breath**: Do prioritize mindful breathing throughout your practice. Deep and controlled breathing can help you relax, reduce stress, and enhance the benefits of chair yoga.

7. **Stay Hydrated**: Make sure you stay hydrated by drinking water both prior to and following your chair yoga session, especially if you're sweating or the practice is longer.

8. **Move Gradually**: Do move through the poses gradually, without rushing. Chair yoga is about slow, controlled movements that promote flexibility and strength over time.

9. **Enjoy the Process**: Do approach chair yoga with a positive mindset and a sense of enjoyment. It's an opportunity to take care of your body and mind.

Don'ts:

1. **Don't Push Beyond Your Limits**: Don't force yourself into poses that feel uncomfortable or painful. Chair yoga is about gentle progression, not pushing yourself to extremes.

2. **Avoid Holding Your Breath**: Don't hold your breath during poses. Maintain a consistent and controlled breathing pattern throughout your session.

3. **Don't Neglect Alignment**: Don't compromise proper alignment for the sake of achieving a deeper stretch. Aligning your body correctly helps prevent strain and injury.

4. **Don't Skip Warm-Up and Cool Down**: Don't skip the warm-up or cool-down phases of your practice. These phases are crucial for preparing your body and preventing muscle soreness.

5. **Avoid Overexertion**: Don't overexert yourself. Chair yoga is designed to be a gentle and accessible form of exercise, so refrain from overexerting yourself.

6. **Avoid Comparisons**: Don't compare yourself to others in the class. Every individual's body is unique, and chair yoga is about personal progress, not competition.

7. **Don't Skip Consultation with Your Doctor**: If you have pre-existing health conditions, don't skip consulting your doctor before starting chair yoga. They can offer precise advice tailored to your individual health status.

8. **Don't Push Through Pain**: If you experience pain during a pose, don't continue with it. Discomfort or pain is a signal to stop and adjust your position.

9. **Avoid Rapid Movements**: Don't rush through the movements. Slow, deliberate movements ensure safety and proper engagement of muscles.

10. **Don't Ignore Safety Guidelines**: Don't overlook safety guidelines and precautions. Following these guidelines ensures a secure and enjoyable chair yoga practice.

By adhering to these dos and don'ts, seniors can experience the benefits of chair yoga while prioritizing their safety, comfort, and well-being. Remember that chair yoga is a supportive and adaptable practice, designed to meet you where you are and enhance your overall quality of life.

Chapter 2:

Getting Started with Chair Yoga

Setting Up Your Space

Establishing a comfortable and secure environment is crucial for the effective practice of chair yoga. By setting up your space thoughtfully, you can ensure a pleasant and enjoyable experience. Here's how to set up your space for chair yoga:

1. **Select a Quiet Area**: Choose a quiet and clutter-free area where you can practice without distractions. This helps you focus on your practice and promotes relaxation.

2. **Clear the Space**: Clear the area of any obstacles or tripping hazards. Make sure there's ample space around your chair for movement and stretching.

3. **Choose a Sturdy Chair**: Use a sturdy and stable chair with a straight back and a flat, non-slip seat. Avoid chairs with wheels or arms that could hinder movement.

4. **Proper Lighting**: Ensure the room is well-lit with natural or artificial light. Good lighting helps you see your movements clearly and prevents strain on your eyes.

5. **Ventilation**: Maintain proper ventilation in the room. Fresh air can enhance your focus and comfort during the practice.

6. **Floor Surface**: If you're standing for any part of your chair yoga practice, ensure the floor surface is non-slip to prevent accidents.

7. **Comfortable Attire**: Wear loose, comfortable clothing that allows for easy movement. Remove any restrictive clothing or accessories that might interfere with your practice.

8. **Props and Accessories**: Gather any props or accessories you plan to use during your practice, such as cushions, blocks, or resistance bands. Having them within reach will help you seamlessly transition between poses.

9. **Water Bottle**: Keep a water bottle nearby to stay hydrated during and after your practice.

10. **Supportive Background**: Choose a supportive and calming background for your practice. You might place a plant, a piece of artwork, or something meaningful within your line of sight.

11. **Timer or Clock**: Have a timer or clock nearby to keep track of your practice time, especially if you're following a guided session with specific time durations.

12. **Meditation or Relaxation Space**: If you plan to incorporate meditation or relaxation into your chair yoga practice, set up a cozy corner with a cushion or blanket where you can sit comfortably afterward.

13. **Personal Touches**: Add personal touches to your space, such as scented candles, calming music, or essential oils, to create an ambiance that promotes relaxation.

Remember that your chair yoga space is a sanctuary for self-care and mindfulness. By creating a welcoming environment, you set the stage for a fulfilling and rejuvenating practice that nourishes your body, mind, and spirit.

Equipment and Props for Chair Yoga

Chair yoga is a versatile practice that can be enhanced with the use of various equipment and props. These props provide support, comfort, and assist in achieving proper alignment during your chair yoga sessions. Here are some common equipment and props used in chair yoga:

1. **Sturdy Chair**: A sturdy chair with a straight back and a flat, non-slip seat is the primary piece of equipment you need for chair yoga. The chair should provide stable support during seated and standing poses.

2. **Cushions and Pillows**: Soft cushions or pillows can be placed on the chair seat or backrest to enhance comfort and support for poses. They can also provide extra cushioning for seated poses.

3. **Yoga Blocks**: These tools can help adapt poses and enhance balance. You can position them beneath your feet, hands, or between your thighs to support correct alignment.

4. **Resistance Bands**: Resistance bands are useful for adding gentle resistance to your movements, which can help improve strength and flexibility. They can be used for both upper and lower body exercises.

5. **Blankets**: Blankets can provide extra cushioning and support for seated poses. They can also be used to cover the chair seat or backrest for added comfort.

6. **Strap or Belt**: A yoga strap or belt can assist in reaching your feet or holding onto your legs during stretches. It's particularly helpful for individuals with limited flexibility.

7. **Small Ball**: A small, soft ball can be used for self-massage and to gently release tension in muscles. It can also be placed between the thighs for inner thigh engagement during certain poses.

8. **Hand Weights**: For those looking to incorporate strength training into their chair yoga practice, lightweight dumbbells or hand weights can be used for resistance exercises.

9. **Timer or Stopwatch**: A timer or stopwatch can help you keep track of the duration of each pose or exercise, ensuring you practice each pose for an appropriate amount of time.

10. **Mirror**: Having a small mirror nearby can help you check your alignment and ensure that you're performing poses correctly. It can be particularly useful for standing poses.

11. **Music or Audio Device**: Calming music or guided meditation recordings can enhance the ambiance of your practice and aid relaxation. Make sure you have an audio device or speakers ready.

12. **Water Bottle**: Staying hydrated during your practice is essential. Keep a water bottle within reach to take sips between poses or exercises.

13. **Yoga Mat**: Although chair yoga is primarily performed while seated or standing with the support of a chair, having a yoga mat on the floor can provide a non-slip surface for your feet and make it more comfortable for certain standing poses.

Breathing Techniques for Relaxation and Mindfulness

Breathing techniques are powerful tools for relaxation and mindfulness. They can aid in soothing the mind, alleviating stress, and fostering inner tranquility. Here are some effective breathing techniques for relaxation and mindfulness:

Deep Abdominal Breathing (Diaphragmatic Breathing):

1. Sit or lie down comfortably.

2. Rest one hand on your chest and the other on your belly.

3. Inhale softly through your nose, allowing your abdomen to rise as your lungs fill with air. Your chest should stay mostly motionless.

4. Gradually exhale through your mouth, softly engaging your abdominal muscles.

5. Practice this profound, rhythmic breathing for a few cycles, paying attention to your abdomen's movement.

6. This technique calms the nervous system and promotes relaxation.

4-7-8 Breathing:

1. Find a comfortable position, either sitting or lying down, and then close your eyes.

2. Inhale gently through your nose, mentally counting up to four.

3. Pause and hold your breath for a duration of seven counts.

4. Fully exhale through your mouth over eight counts, producing a whoosh-like sound.

5. Repeat this cycle three more times for a total of four breaths.

6. This method can aid in alleviating anxiety and fostering relaxation.

Box Breathing (4-4-4-4):

1. Find a comfortable seated position.

2. Inhale quietly through your nose to a count of four.

3. Take a breath and hold it for a count of four.

4. Gently exhale through your mouth, counting to four as you release the breath.

5. Pause and hold your breath for another count of four.

6. Repeat this cycle for several rounds.

7. Box breathing helps regulate your breath and brings a sense of calm.

Alternate Nostril Breathing (Nadi Shodhana):

1. Find a comfortable seating position, ensuring your spine is erect.

2. Utilize your right thumb to block your right nostril, then take a breath in through the left nostril.

3. Seal your left nostril using your right ring finger, open your right nostril, and breathe out from the right side.

4. Draw a breath in through the right nostril, then shut it with your thumb, and breathe out from the left nostril.

5. This sequence marks one full cycle. Continue for multiple rounds.

6. Nadi Shodhana harmonizes the brain's left and right regions, aiding in mental clarity and calmness.

Mindful Breathing:

1. Find a comfortable position, either sitting or lying down, and then close your eyes.

2. Bring your attention to your breath without attempting to change it.

3. Observe the natural rhythm of your breath, the rise and fall of your chest or abdomen, and the sensation of the breath entering and leaving your nostrils.

4. If you find that your attention has wandered, bring it back to focusing on your breath in a gentle way.

5. Practice mindfulness of your breath for a few minutes to quiet the mind and increase present-moment awareness.

Counted Breath Meditation:

6. Sit in a comfortable position.

7. Breathe in gently through your nose, counting to four.

8. Breathe out through your mouth, counting up to six.

9. Repeat this cycle for several minutes, gradually extending the exhalation count to eight or ten.

10. This practice encourages relaxation and mental clarity.

These breathing techniques can be practiced individually or combined, depending on your preferences and needs. Consistent application of these methods can aid in stress management, anxiety reduction, and foster heightened mindfulness and overall well-being in everyday living.

Chapter 3:

Seated Warm-Up Exercises

A seated warm-up exercise before engaging in chair yoga is of paramount importance, especially for seniors. This initial phase serves as a critical preparatory step to ensure the safety, efficacy, and overall enjoyment of the chair yoga practice tailored for older adults.

A seated warm-up exercise is vital for injury prevention. Seniors often have reduced flexibility and joint mobility, making it essential to ease into physical activity. The gentle movements involved in a warm-up help lubricate joints, enhance blood flow to muscles, and prepare the body for more complex chair yoga poses. By doing so, it significantly reduces the risk of strains, sprains, or discomfort during the yoga session.

Moreover, the seated warm-up fosters a mindful and calming atmosphere. It encourages seniors to synchronize their breath with their movements, focusing their attention on the present moment. This mental preparation enhances the meditative aspect of chair yoga, leading to relaxation, stress reduction, and improved mental clarity.

The warm-up serves as a check-in with the body, highlighting any areas of tension or discomfort. Seniors can use this newfound awareness to adapt their practice accordingly, ensuring it remains safe and tailored to their unique needs.

The seated warm-up exercise is the cornerstone of a safe, effective, and holistic chair yoga practice for seniors. It addresses physical and mental well-being, reduces the risk of injury, and deepens the connection to the practice, making it an indispensable component of senior wellness through yoga.

Neck Tilts

Seated neck tilts are a gentle warm-up exercise that helps relieve tension and stiffness in the neck and upper back. This exercise promotes flexibility in the neck and can be especially beneficial for seniors who may experience neck discomfort or limited range of motion.

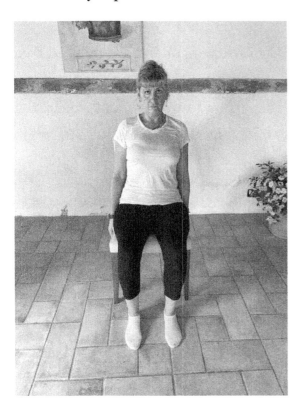 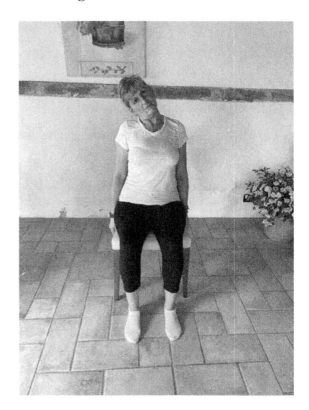

Instructions:

1. Position yourself upright in a stable chair, ensuring your feet are firmly on the ground.

2. Move your head to the right in small increments, bringing your right ear closer to your right shoulder as you do so.

3. Maintain the stretch for 15 to 20 secs, and you should feel a light stretch over the left side of your neck.

4. Bring your head back to the middle of your body.

5. Perform the same movement on the left side, this time pushing your left ear closer to your left shoulder.

6. Hold for 15-20 seconds.

7. Repeat this motion 2-3 times on each side.

Arm Raises

Seated arm raises are an excellent warm-up exercise for seniors that help improve shoulder flexibility and posture. This activity is easy on the joints and can be conveniently performed while sitting.

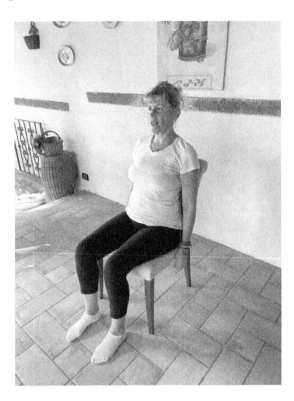 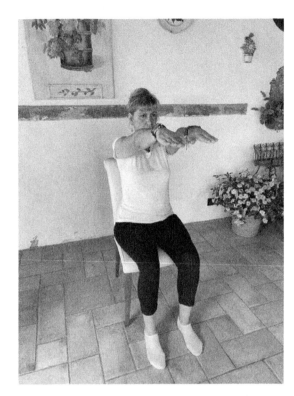

Instructions:

1. Position yourself upright, ensuring your feet are firmly on the ground and your arms are relaxed by your sides.

2. Slowly raise both arms in front of you, keeping them straight.

3. Continue raising your arms until they are at shoulder level.

4. Hold for a couple of secs.

5. Lower your arms back to your sides.

6. Repeat this motion 10-15 times.

Seated Leg Extensions

Seated leg extensions are an excellent way to warm up the muscles in your thighs and improve flexibility in your lower body. This exercise can also help increase circulation to the legs.

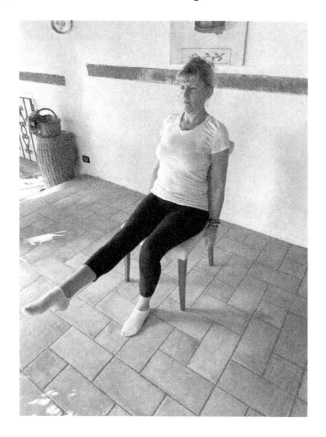

Instructions:

1. Sit upright, ensuring your feet are firmly planted on the ground.

2. Stretch your right leg in front of you in a straight line while maintaining your foot in a flexed position.

3. Maintain this position for a couple of secs.

4. Bring your right foot back down to the ground.

5. Repeat the previous step with your left leg.

6. Continue alternating between right and left legs.

7. Perform 10-15 extensions on each leg.

8. For added challenge, you can use ankle weights.

Seated Knee Lifts

Seated knee lifts are an excellent warm-up exercise to engage the abdominal muscles, increase hip flexibility, and improve circulation in the lower extremities. This activity is particularly advantageous for the elderly since it can be done while seated, accommodating those with restricted mobility.

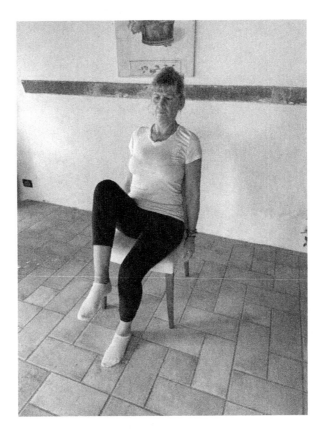

Instructions:

1. Sit upright, ensuring your feet are firmly planted on the ground.

2. Hold onto the sides of your chair for support.

3. Lift your right knee as high as you can, bringing it towards your chest.

4. Hold for a few seconds.

5. Lower your right foot back to the floor.

6. Repeat with your left knee.

7. Continue alternating between right and left knees.

8. Perform 10-15 knee lifts on each leg.

Shoulder Rolls

Shoulder rolls are a simple yet effective seated warm-up exercise that helps improve shoulder mobility and reduce tension in the upper back and shoulders. This exercise can be especially beneficial for seniors who may experience stiffness in the upper body.

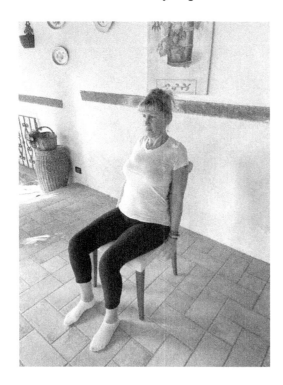 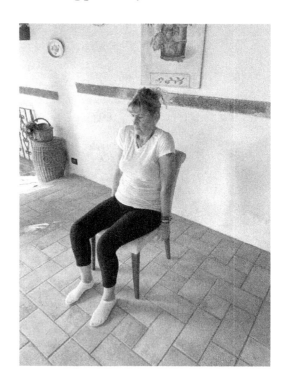

Instructions:

1. Maintain an upright posture with your arms relaxed by your sides.

2. Gently roll your shoulders forward in a circular motion, making small circles.

3. Complete 10-15 forward rolls.

4. Reverse the motion, rolling your shoulders backward in small circles.

5. Complete 10-15 backward rolls.

6. Repeat this cycle 2-3 times.

Ankle Rotations

Ankle rotations are a seated warm-up exercise that helps improve ankle flexibility and circulation in the lower legs. This activity is especially beneficial for seniors who may experience stiffness or discomfort in their ankles.

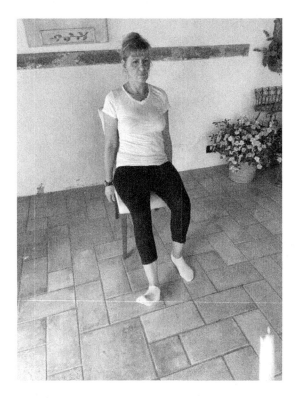 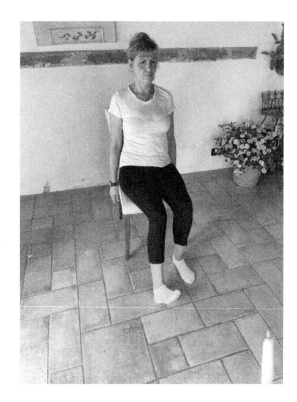

Instructions:

1. Sit upright, ensuring your feet are firmly planted on the ground.

2. Lift your right foot slightly off the ground.

3. Begin making slow, circular motions with your right ankle, rotating it clockwise.

4. Perform 10-15 clockwise rotations.

5. Reverse the direction, rotating your right ankle counterclockwise for 10-15 rotations.

6. Lower your right foot to the floor.

7. Repeat the same process with your left ankle.

8. Perform 2-3 sets on each ankle.

Seated Chest Opener

The Seated Chest Opener is an excellent exercise for seniors to counteract the effects of slouching and improve chest and shoulder mobility.

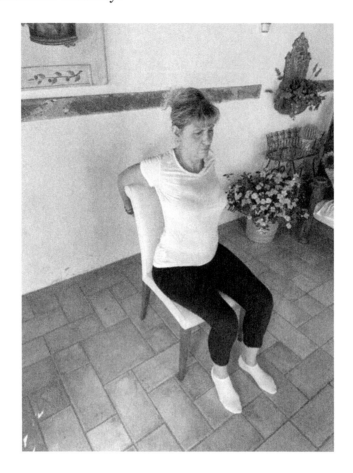

Instructions:

1. Sit upright, ensuring your feet are firmly planted on the ground.

2. Put your hands behind your back and clasp them together.

3. Raise your chest and gently bring your shoulder blades closer together while maintaining a neutral spine.

4. Maintain this position for 15 to 20 secs as you feel a stretch throughout your chest and shoulders.

5. Release and relax.

6. Repeat the stretch 2-3 times.

Seated Marching

Seated marching is an excellent warm-up exercise for seniors to improve circulation, engage the leg muscles, and gently warm up the lower body. It's also a low-impact exercise, making it suitable for individuals with various fitness levels.

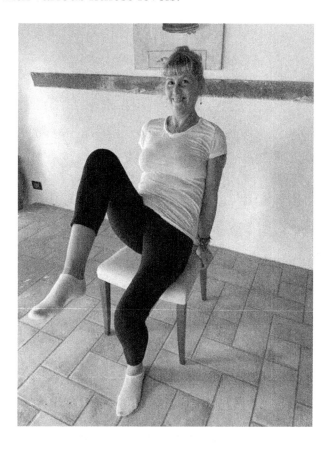

Instructions:

1. Sit upright, ensuring your feet are firmly planted on the ground.

2. Lift your right knee as high as you comfortably can while keeping your left foot on the ground.

3. Lower your right foot back to the floor.

4. Do the same action with your left knee as you did with your right knee.

5. Pretend that you are marching in place and continue to switch back and forth among your right and left knees.

6. March for 1-2 minutes.

Seated Wrist and Finger Flexibility

Seated wrist and finger flexibility exercises are great for seniors as they help improve hand mobility and reduce stiffness, which can be especially beneficial for those who may have arthritis or other hand-related issues.

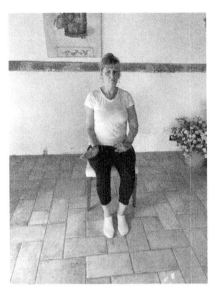 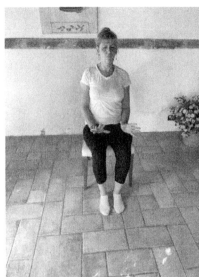 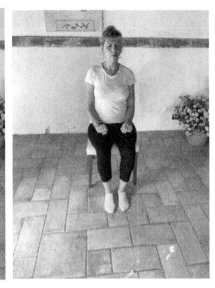

Instructions:

1. Sit upright, placing your hands gently on your thighs.

2. Begin by making slow circles with your wrists, rotating them clockwise for 10-15 seconds.

3. Reverse the direction, rotating your wrists counterclockwise for 10-15 seconds.

4. Next, extend your fingers wide apart and then make a fist.

5. Repeat the open-and-close motion with your fingers for 10-15 seconds.

6. Shake out your hands to release any tension.

7. Repeat both exercises 2-3 times.

Seated Diaphragmatic Breathing

Seated diaphragmatic breathing is an excellent warm-up exercise for seniors, as it helps relax the body, reduce stress, and improve lung function. It's a calming exercise that can prepare the body for more active movements and can be done from the comfort of a chair.

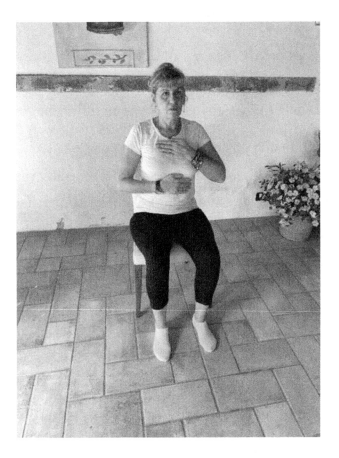

Instructions:

1. Sit upright, ensuring your feet are firmly planted on the ground.

2. Put your hands on your abdomen.

3. Inhale deeply and calmly through your nose, letting your belly rise as your lungs take in air.

4. Release your breath slowly through your mouth, allowing your abdomen to fall.

5. Pay attention to the upward and downward movement of your abdomen with each deep breath.

6. Continue this deep breathing for 1-2 minutes.

7. This exercise can also be combined with other seated warm-up exercises to enhance relaxation and focus.

Chapter 4:

Chair Yoga for Balance and Posture

As individuals age, the risk of balance issues and posture imbalances becomes more prevalent, leading to a higher susceptibility to falls and discomfort. Chair yoga offers a gentle and effective approach to address these concerns, ensuring seniors can fully reap the benefits of their practice.

By emphasizing balance-enhancing poses and postural awareness, chair yoga cultivates stability, thereby reducing the likelihood of falls. It targets the muscles responsible for maintaining equilibrium, strengthening them gradually and safely. Additionally, chair yoga heightens proprioception – the body's awareness of its position in space – which is vital for balance control.

Moreover, chair yoga encourages the alignment of the spine and promotes proper posture. It combats the tendency to slouch or slump that often accompanies aging. Through mindful engagement in various poses, seniors develop an improved awareness of their body alignment, which extends beyond the practice and becomes ingrained in daily activities.

Prioritizing balance and posture through chair yoga not only fosters physical well-being but also enhances self-confidence and independence. With a foundation of stability and proper alignment, seniors can embark on their chair yoga exercises with greater comfort and security, embracing the holistic benefits of improved balance, enhanced posture, and overall vitality.

Seated Spinal Twist (Ardha Matsyendrasana)

The Seated Spinal Twist is a modified version of the classic yoga pose, Ardha Matsyendrasana, designed precisely for seniors & those with restricted mobility. This pose helps improve spinal flexibility, increase circulation to the spine, and enhance balance, all while sitting comfortably in a chair.

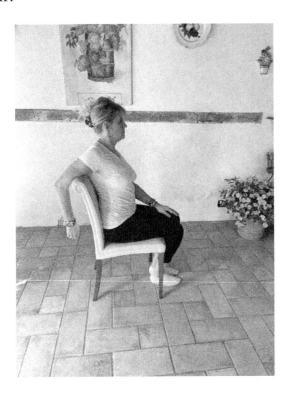 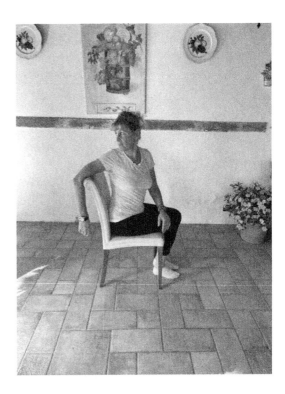

Instructions:

1. Place both of your feet flat on the floor and bring your knees close as you sit.

2. Put your left hand on your right knee and your right arm on the backrest of the chair.

3. Take a deep breath in, stretch your spine, and then release while gradually rotating to the right.

4. Maintain this position for 20 to 30 secs while taking deep breaths, and then transfer sides.

Seated Warrior I

Seated Warrior I is a modified version of the traditional Warrior I pose, adapted for seniors to improve balance and posture while seated in a chair. This pose strengthens the legs, stretches the spine, and promotes better posture.

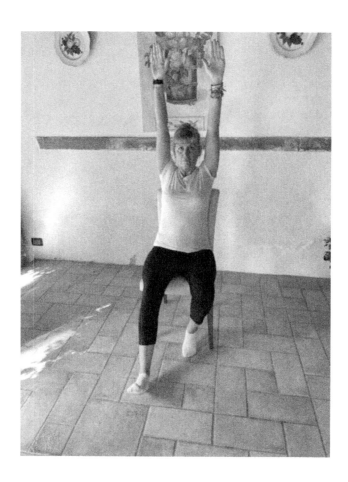

Instructions:

1. Maintain an upright seated posture with your feet positioned at hip-width apart.

2. Extend your right leg straight out in front of you, toes pointing up.

3. Gently bend your left knee and nestle your left foot beneath the chair.

4. Inhale, reach your arms overhead, keeping your spine straight.

5. Hold for 20-30 seconds, then switch sides.

Seated Mountain Pose (Tadasana)

Seated Mountain Pose is a foundational yoga posture that helps seniors improve their balance, posture, and overall body awareness while sitting comfortably in a chair. This pose promotes a sense of groundedness and alignment, making it an excellent starting point for any chair yoga routine.

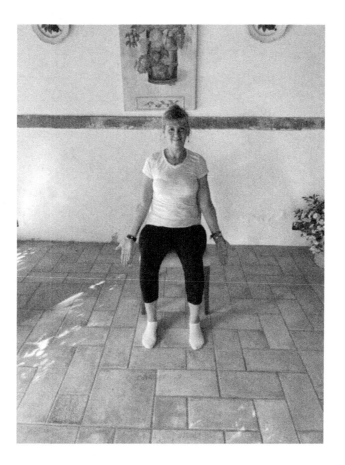

Instructions:

1. Sit upright in the chair, ensuring your feet are firmly planted on the ground and spaced hip-width apart.

2. Let your arms to rest comfortably by your sides, with palms turned forward.

3. Close your eyes and take deep breaths for 1-2 minutes, feeling grounded and centered.

Seated Cat-Cow Stretch

The Seated Cat-Cow Stretch is a gentle chair yoga exercise designed to improve spinal flexibility, enhance posture, and alleviate tension in the back. It's particularly beneficial for seniors who may experience stiffness in their spine and want to maintain or regain mobility.

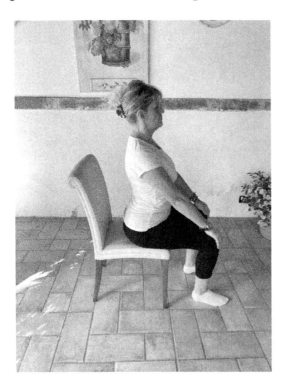 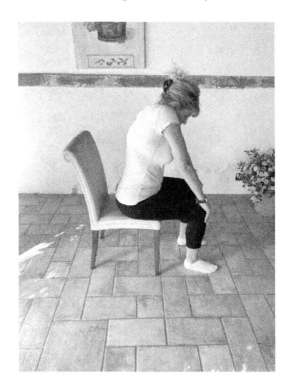

Instructions:

1. Sit up straight in the chair.

2. Breathe in, curve your spine outward, and raise your chest (Cow Pose).

3. Exhale, round your back, tuck your chin (Cat Pose).

4. Repeat this movement for 1-2 minutes, coordinating breath with movement.

Seated Forward Fold (Paschimottanasana)

The Seated Forward Fold is a gentle stretch that targets the spine, hamstrings, and lower back. It helps to improve posture by lengthening the spine & reducing tension in the lower back.

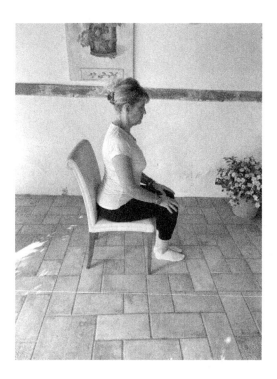 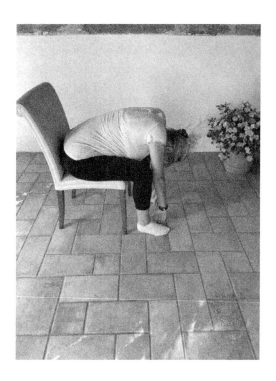

Instructions:

1. Sit with your feet flat on the floor.

2. Inhale, lengthen your spine, and exhale as you gently fold forward from your hips.

3. Reach your hands towards your feet or ankles, maintaining your back as straight as probable.

4. Hold for 20-30 seconds while breathing deeply.

Seated Tree Pose (Vrksasana)

Seated Tree Pose is a modified version of the classic Tree Pose (Vrksasana) adapted for seniors who may have difficulty standing for extended periods. This pose is excellent for enhancing balance, posture, and leg strength. It also encourages mental focus and concentration.

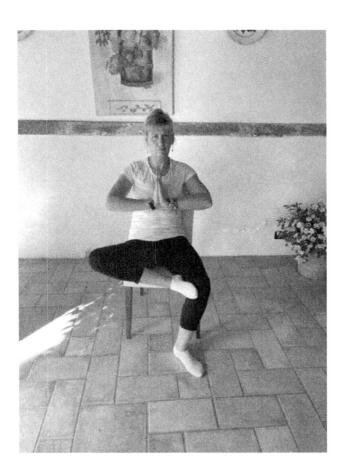

Instructions:

1. Sit upright, ensuring your feet are firmly planted on the ground.

2. Elevate your right foot and position it on the inner thigh of your left leg, ensuring the toes are pointing downward.

3. Press your hands together in front of your chest.

4. Hold for 20-30 secs, then switch sides.

Chair Yoga Half-Split Pose

The half-split pose is slightly different. Instead of remaining seated, you stand up, face your chair and use it for support. This pose targets proprioception, which is your ability to recognize your body's movements in space and improve balance. Proprioception is usually affected by neurological disorders such as Alzheimer's, strokes, Parkinson's, and multiple sclerosis, to mention a few.

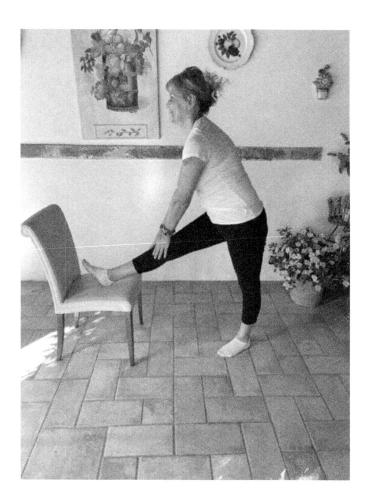

Instructions:

1. Stand and face your chair. Maintain an arms-length distance. If you have balance issues, turn your chair around to a 90° angle.

2. Lift your right foot and step on the chair's sitting area. This leaves your left foot on the ground, which is currently supporting your body's entire weight.

3. Straighten your right foot and ensure it rests on the chair's sitting area with your heel, toes pointing upwards.

4. You have two options: (1) you can work on the balance of your left leg in this position, or (2) put your hands on your elevated leg and fold forward.

5. For that extra stretch at the back of your leg, move your foot's toes towards you and away from you a few times while ensuring the right foot still rests on its heel. Count a few breaths and return your upper body back to a straight standing position.

6. Now change legs, place your left foot on the chair, and repeat the process.

Seated Warrior III

A significant amount of abdominal control and buttock strength are required for the Warrior III chair position. Regardless, the practice of this position is quite relaxing and pleasurable. This is the optimal posture for boosting stamina and strength in the legs, core, and back, as well as promoting attention, which makes it great to enhance metabolism.

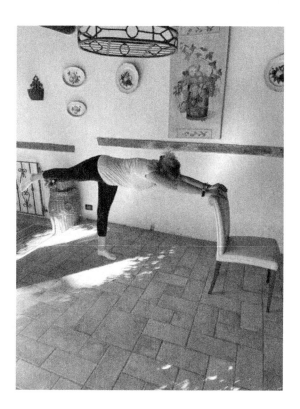 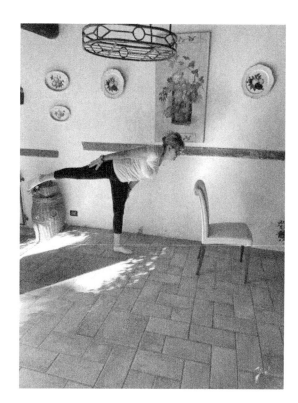

Instructions:

1. To get started, you should first stand in the back of your chair. Walk backwards while keeping your hands on the very top of the chair back till your upper body is at a right angle to the ground.

2. Extend your right leg behind you. Bring your hips into a level position, as if you were going to put a teacup on your lower back.

3. Extend a stick from the bottom of your heel to the top of your head. If you think that you're prepared, you can put your balance to the test by releasing your grip on the chair and lowering your arms to your sides.

4. Hold every side for anywhere between five and eight breaths.

Seated Hamstring Stretch

This pose helps stretch calves and hamstrings and activates core abdominal muscles, which can help to promote good balance. To perform this pose, you will require a yoga strap or a belt to use as a prop.

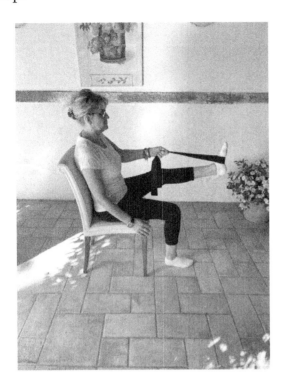 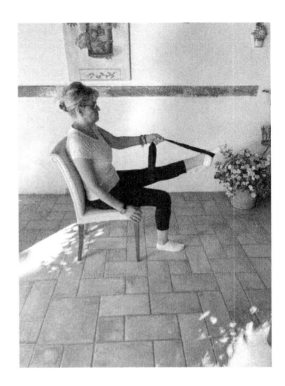

Instructions:

1. Make a loop with a belt or strap and hook it around your left foot. Hold the ends of the strap in your left hand. During this stretch, you can hold the edge of the chair with your right hand for extra support if needed.

2. Begin with maintaining your back as straight as feasible, begin to straighten your left leg and lift it off the ground. You can keep a bend in your knee if it is more comfortable.

3. While holding the pose, perform a few repetitions of pointing and flexing your foot to engage your calf muscles. This will help to encourage proper circulation.

4. Hold the stretch for 30 seconds.

5. Lower your left foot back to the floor and release the strap.

6. Rest for one minute, and then repeat the exercise with your right leg.

7. Repeat the stretch three to five times on each leg.

8. For an extra challenge, loosen the strap a little so that you are using your hip flexor muscles to keep your leg lifted.

Chapter 5:

Chair Yoga for Lower Body Mobility and Strength

Chair yoga holds profound importance for seniors in enhancing lower body mobility and strength. As individuals age, maintaining these vital aspects of physical well-being becomes increasingly crucial for overall health and independence. Chair yoga offers a safe and accessible means to address these needs.

Lower body mobility is crucial for daily activities like standing, walking, and climbing stairs. Chair yoga's gentle movements and stretches specifically target the lower body, helping to improve flexibility in the hips, knees, and ankles. This enhanced range of motion translates into increased ease in performing daily tasks and a reduced risk of falls.

Chair yoga strengthens the lower body muscles, comprising the quadriceps, hamstrings, and calf muscles. These muscles are essential for stability and balance. By engaging in chair yoga regularly, seniors can build and maintain strength in these areas, providing greater support for their body weight and reducing the risk of muscle atrophy.

Moreover, chair yoga fosters improved posture, alignment, and body awareness, which are crucial for preventing common age-related issues such as lower back pain and joint stiffness. The incorporation of weight-bearing exercises in chair yoga also helps preserve bone density, reducing the risk of osteoporosis.

Chair yoga serves as an invaluable tool for seniors to enhance lower body mobility and strength, promoting not only physical well-being but also a sense of confidence and independence in their daily lives.

Seated Spinal Twist II

This twisting pose relieves lower back pain, encourages spinal mobility, and simultaneously relaxes and invigorates. In addition, twisting in this manner can help to tone your belly, massage internal organs, and promote good digestion. It is often performed towards the end of a routine after the muscles have been warmed up and worked a little bit.

The spinal twist movement works all muscle groups: glutes, hips, abdominals, obliques, lower back, mid-back, shoulders, and chest.

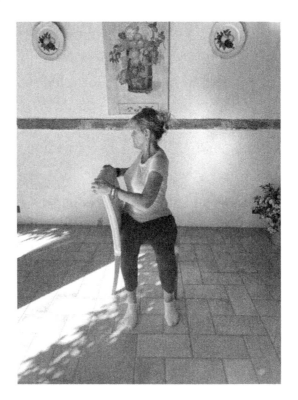

Instructions:

1. Sit sideways on your chair. Face to the right with your right arm against the chair's back and your feet on the floor.

2. Inhale and sit tall, elongating the spine.

3. As you exhale, rotate your upper body to the right. Grab the back of the chair with both hands, twisting your spine.

4. Remain in this position for 30 seconds.

5. Release your hands and move back to the starting position.

6. Rotate on the chair so that you are facing the left. Repeat the stretch to the left.

7. Repeat three to five times on each side.

Seated Hip Openers

Seated hip openers in chair yoga can be an effective way to improve lower body mobility and strength, especially for individuals who may have difficulty with traditional yoga poses due to physical limitations.

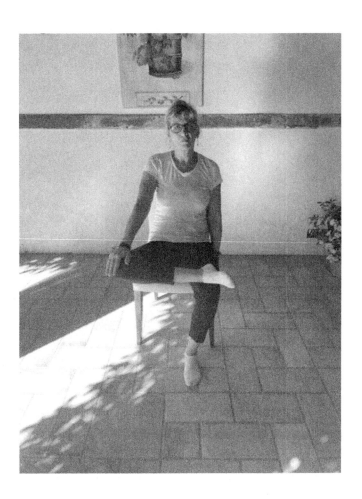

Instructions:

1. Place the right ankle over the left knee.

2. Let the right knee relax to the side as you keep the foot flexed.

3. As you breathe in, sit up straight, and as you breathe out, enjoy stretching that area of your body.

4. You can considerably extend the stretch by laying your right hand on your right knee and exerting light pressure in this position. This will allow you to further enhance the stretch.

5. Keep your back flat and twist as you lean forward using your hips.

6. Stay in this position for three to five breaths and repeat on the other side.

Seated Butterfly Pose

The Butterfly pose will help loosen your hips, lower back, and thighs. This movement can also improve circulation throughout the body. To do this pose, you will need a cushion, yoga block, or stack of books to rest your feet on and raise your knees slightly.

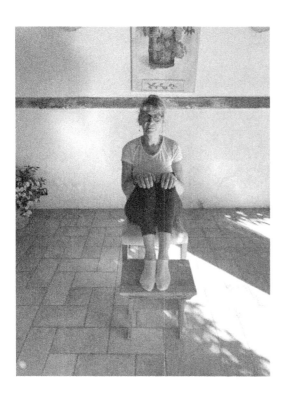 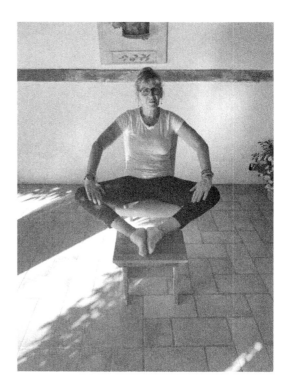

Instructions:

1. Sit comfortably in a chair with your feet propped up on a cushion or other stable block. Start with a height of two to three inches, and then raise the height if you wish.

2. With your hands on your knees and your knees together, inhale deeply.

3. Exhale and allow your knees to separate and fall towards the floor. Don't force them, just allow them to move on their own.

4. Inhale deeply, and then with an exhale push lightly on your knees to deepen the stretch a little bit more.

Seated Wide-Legged Forward Bend Pose

The Seated Wide-Legged Forward Bend Pose is a modified yoga pose that can be performed using a chair. It's an excellent option for individuals with limited mobility or those who find it challenging to perform traditional yoga poses on the floor. This pose helps improve lower body mobility and strength while providing a gentle stretch for the hamstrings and lower back.

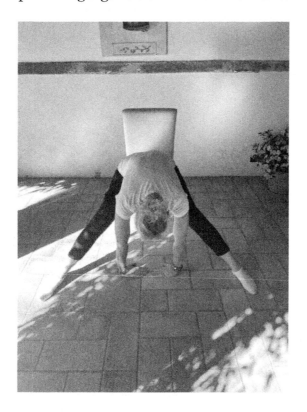

Instructions:

1. Position yourself so that you are seated in the exact middle of your chair and extend your legs out to the side. You can either put your feet in a flat position on the ground or you can raise your toes whilst driving your heels into the ground.

2. Ensure that you are sitting in a comfortable position by pressing the bones of your seat into the chair and by ensuring that your feet and knees are facing the same direction.

3. Take a long, deep breath in, and as you let it out, lean forward from the hips and press your weight into the soles of your feet. Push your body forward till your hand is in contact with the floor or the blocks (if you are using them).

4. Lean forward and get as low as you can while still maintaining your comfort level. Take a moment to relax here, pressing your body into your palms. You are able to stretch the legs outward if you choose, but before you do so, ensure that you are as stable and at ease as is humanly feasible.

5. To exit the pose, begin to slowly walk your way up to a standing position. To prevent vertigo or dizziness, you should avoid rushing at all costs.

Seated Half Pigeon Pose

Seated Half Pigeon Pose in chair yoga is a modified version of the traditional Pigeon Pose (Eka Pada Rajakapotasana) that helps improve lower body mobility and strength while accommodating individuals with limited flexibility or mobility. This pose primarily targets the hips, thighs, and lower back.

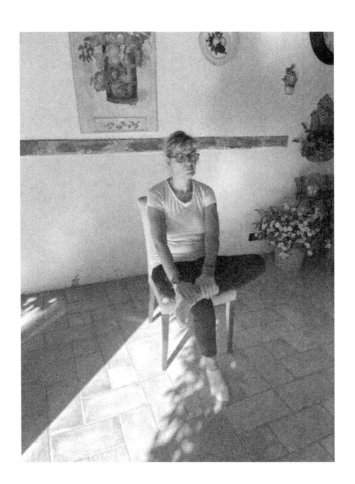

Instructions:

1. Start by comfortably sitting down with your arms on your knees or thighs.

2. Take a deep breath before holding your left ankle with both hands.

3. Slowly lift your left leg sideways towards your right knee as you breathe out.

4. Place your left ankle to rest on your right thigh or knee, then remain in that position for about 20 seconds.

5. Return your leg to its original position before repeating the same procedure with your right leg.

Seated Knee to Forehead Bend Pose

The Seated Knee to Forehead Bend Pose in chair yoga is a great exercise for improving lower body mobility and strength. This posture primarily focuses on stretching the hamstrings, lower back, and hip flexors, all while engaging the core muscles.

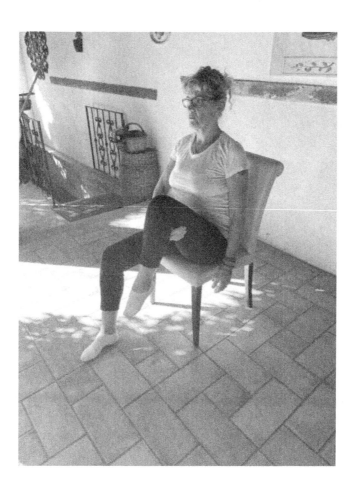

Instructions:

1. Sit firmly on your chair; lengthen your spine, with feet firmly on the floor. Take a deep breath in and shift your pelvis slightly backward.

2. Tuck your chin in, round your back, and raise your left knee towards your forehead. Use your right hand to support the lift from under the knee.

3. Raise your knee as far as you can comfortably manage, and hold the position for 2-3 breaths. Do not attempt to push your knee further up if this action feels strained or painful. Your knee does not necessarily have to go all the way up to meet your forehead.

4. Lower your left knee slowly back to the floor and repeat the same process with your right knee, this time using your left hand as support.

5. Repeat the stretch at least 4-5 times on each knee.

Seated Figure-Four Stretch

Many people who sit for large portions of their days will have lower back pain. One of the best ways to combat and prevent this is to stretch out the gluteus muscles and the hips. This stretch will help relieve any lower back tension that you are feeling and the tension surrounding the sacrum. In addition, any people who feel pain in the sciatic nerve will find relief by doing the figure 4 stretch.

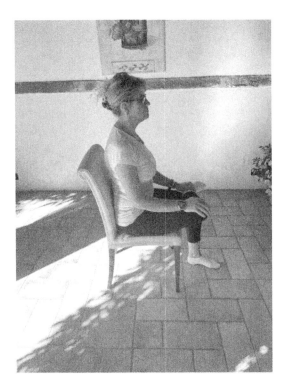 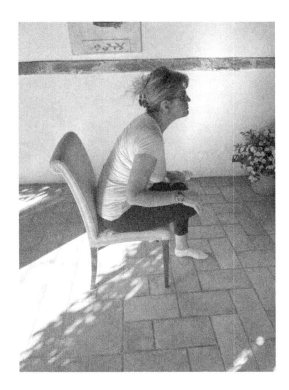

Instructions:

1. Find a comfortable position in your chair and maintain a straight spine while placing both feet firmly on the floor.

2. Bend your right leg, positioning the ankle on your left thigh.

3. Flex your right foot.

4. Put your left hand on your right heel and your right hand on your right thigh.

5. While maintaining a straight back, pivot forward at the hips over your bent leg.

6. Hold this position for five breaths, then gradually ease out of the pose.

7. Repeat with the left leg and then repeat five times on each side.

If this stretch is either too difficult or too easy for you, try changing the angle you bend your knee. If you would like to increase the stretch, bend your knee more. Do not bend your knee as much if you want less of a stretch.

Seated Cobbler's Pose

Seated Cobbler's Pose is a yoga pose that can be adapted for chair yoga to improve lower body mobility and strength while seated. This pose primarily targets the hips, groin, and lower back.

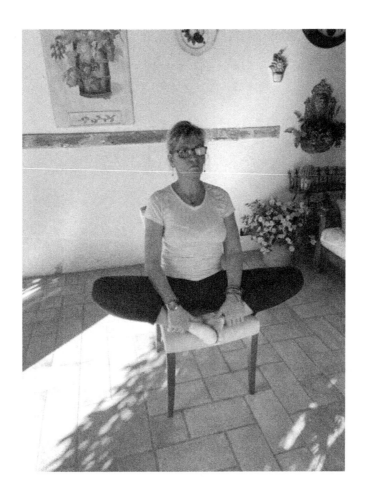

Instructions:

1. Take up the mountain pose, then stretch both legs straight on the floor to rest on your heels.

2. Fold your left leg, lift it up with your hand and place it on the chair's base—ensure you use a chair with a wide sitting area for this pose. Lift your right leg and place it, knee bent, lying on the sitting area of your chair. Now you are seated with the soles of the feet together.

3. Both knees should be lying flat on your chair's sitting area. However, do not attempt to push or force them down with your hands if they are not. Allow them to remain at their lowest natural position.

4. Hold this position for as long as you can without straining. Also, avoid rounding your back or shoulders; they should remain upright and at ease.

Seated Hero's Pose or Virasana

Seated Hero's Pose (Virasana) is a yoga pose that can be adapted for chair yoga to improve lower body mobility and strength. This variation is particularly useful for individuals who may have difficulty sitting on the floor due to flexibility or mobility issues.

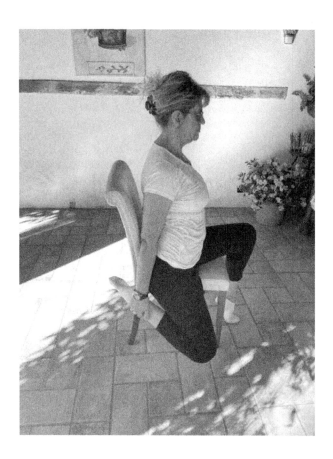

Instructions:

1. Move to the edge of your chair such that your right leg is 'hanging' off on one side of the seat. Stabilize yourself by using your left hand to hold on to the chair.

2. Lean towards the left side, and at the same time, bend your right knee while holding your foot with your right hand. You can make the exercise easier by using a strap or belt to loop your foot.

3. Slowly pull your foot behind, towards your glute. The point is to stretch the front part of your thigh and feel the resultant pull.

4. If you feel some form of sensation on your knee, you have pulled your foot too far back; release your hold slowly until the sensations disappear.

5. Repeat the above process with your left leg and perform around five repetitions for each leg.

Chapter 6:

Chair Yoga for Upper Body Mobility and Strength

As we age, maintaining upper body strength and flexibility becomes increasingly important for daily functioning and independence. Chair yoga provides a safe and accessible way for seniors to achieve and sustain these essential attributes.

Chair yoga exercises specifically target a variety of muscle groups in the upper body, encompassing the arms, shoulders, and chest. Through gentle and deliberate movements and stretches, these exercises enhance muscle tone and strength. This can be particularly valuable in preventing muscle atrophy and lowering the risk of falls or injuries. This newfound strength enables seniors to perform daily tasks with greater ease and confidence.

Moreover, chair yoga enhances upper body mobility by promoting joint flexibility and range of motion. Seniors often experience stiffness in the shoulders and neck, which can lead to discomfort and restricted movement. Chair yoga's gentle stretches and rotations alleviate tension in these areas, resulting in increased mobility and reduced discomfort.

Beyond the physical benefits, chair yoga fosters mental well-being. It encourages mindfulness through coordinated breath and movement, reducing stress and anxiety. This, in turn, can have a positive impact on posture and upper body comfort, as stress-induced tension often accumulates in these regions.

Seated Half Lotus Pose

Seated Half Lotus Pose is a classic yoga pose that involves sitting with one foot on top of the opposite thigh. However, when practicing chair yoga, you'll need to make modifications to perform this pose while sitting in a chair. This modified pose can help improve upper body mobility and strength.

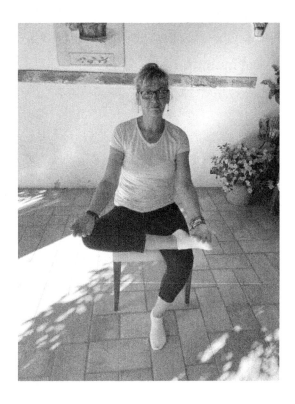

Instructions:

1. Place both feet firmly on the floor, keeping them parallel to one another and hip-distance apart, and sit up straight in the chair.

2. Cross your right ankle across your left leg, and then pull your right knee to the side while maintaining the cross.

3. With your hands at ease and your palms pointing up, put your right hand on your right knee and your left hand on your right foot. Keep your right hand on your right knee.

4. Maintain a tall and upright seated position, close your eyes, and take deeper breaths.

5. Draw your attention inward with your mind and concentrate on your breathing while you slowly and deeply inhale through your nose.

6. Stay in this position and take 15 to 25 slow, deep breaths.

7. Once you are prepared, slowly and softly bring yourself to open your eyes, uncross your leg, and release your hands.

8. On the other side, repeat steps 2 through 7 in the same order as before.

Downward-Facing Dog Pose

The Downward-Facing Dog Pose is a classic yoga pose that provides a great stretch and strength-building exercise for the upper body, particularly the shoulders, arms, and upper back. However, it can be challenging for some individuals to perform, especially if they have limited mobility or strength in their upper body. Chair yoga modifications can make this pose accessible and effective for those with physical limitations.

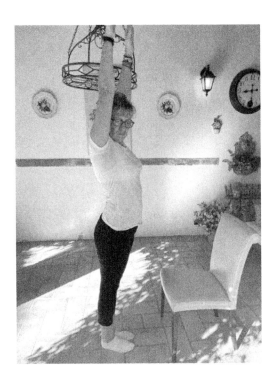 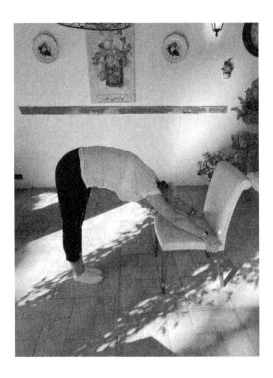

Instructions:

1. Position yourself so that your body is facing the chair seat as you stand in front of it. You ought to maintain a space of approximately two feet between yourself and the chair.

2. While still standing, take a deep breath and raise your arms above your head. Now let out an exhalation as you move forward, leaning forward from the hips, and reaching forward with extended arms to grab the chair that is in front of you.

3. Take a deep breath in and relax your body while it is still in contact with the chair. Make use of the chair as a support while you stretch out your arms, shoulders, upper back, and spine.

4. Hold this position for the duration of six breaths, gradually delving further into the stretch with each outgoing breath.

5. Relax your body and come back to standing position.

Seated Eagle Pose with Arm Raise

The Seated Eagle Pose with Arm Raise is a chair yoga pose that can help improve upper body mobility and strength. This posture is an adapted variation of the conventional Eagle Pose and is appropriate for individuals who might encounter limited mobility or balance challenges.

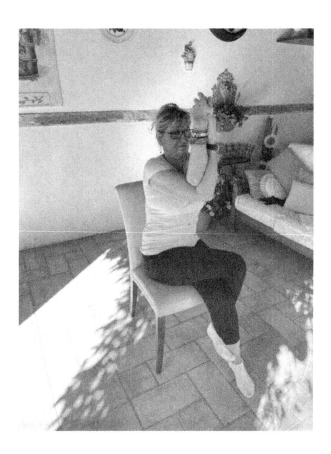

Instructions:

1. Sit with your feet hip-distance apart, firmly on the floor. Remember to always keep your back straight.

2. Cross your right leg over your left leg so that the knees are close together. If mobility allows, move your left foot slightly forward and wrap your right toes around your left leg. Take your arms out at shoulder height.

3. Cross your left elbow over your right elbow and keep your arms at an angle of 90 degrees, with your fingers pointing towards the ceiling. Bend your elbows then bring your palms together.

4. Lift your elbows as you spread your shoulders. Inhale as you do this and hold the position for at least five seconds. Exhale and release, repeating in the other direction.

Seated Raised Hands Pose

Seated Raised Hands Pose, also known as Urdhva Hastasana, is a yoga pose that can be adapted for chair yoga to improve upper body mobility and strength. Chair yoga offers a fantastic choice for individuals with restricted mobility or those in need of additional support.

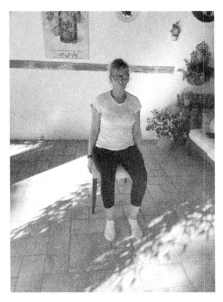 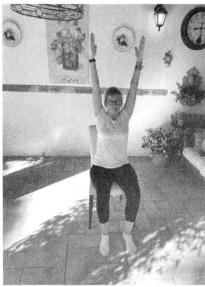 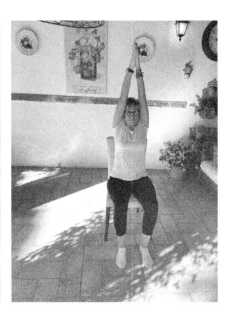

Instructions:

1. Sit in a mountain pose and then methodically raise your arms straight outwards to your side. Next, lift them both upwards above your head, with your elbows straight.

2. Your arms should be parallel; if possible, bring your palms together over your head and ensure you do not hunch your shoulders. If you let your palms remain apart, they should face each other.

3. When you raise your arms, your shoulders will automatically move up. Slide them down away from your ears to allow your collar bones to broaden from the pose. If you feel your rib cage is being pulled apart or jutting forward, knit your shoulders back together.

4. With your arms still overhead, gently pull your navel towards your spine, ensuring your chest remains lifted.

5. Hold this pose for 20-30 seconds, and then lower your arms by your side to relax. You can perform the workout 5-10 more times.

Seated Cobra Pose

The Seated Cobra Pose is a modified yoga pose that can be performed using a chair, making it accessible for individuals with limited mobility or those who have difficulty getting down on the floor. It primarily targets the upper body, including the chest, shoulders, and upper back, to improve mobility and strength.

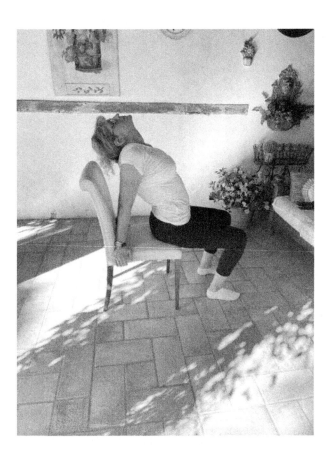

Instructions:

1. Place your hands on the chair's back while you inhale. As you exhale, shift your hips forward.

2. Inhale, then extend your arms, chest, and spine by bending them backward.

3. Exhale and tilt your head back.

4. Take this backbend and hold it in the Cobra Pose Chair for eight breaths while inhaling and exhaling.

5. Release tension by inhaling and exhaling.

Upward Facing Dog Pose With Chair

Upward Facing Dog Pose, also known as Urdhva Mukha Svanasana, is a classic yoga pose that helps improve upper body mobility and strength. However, it can be challenging for some individuals, especially those with limited mobility or strength. Using a chair as a prop can make this pose more accessible.

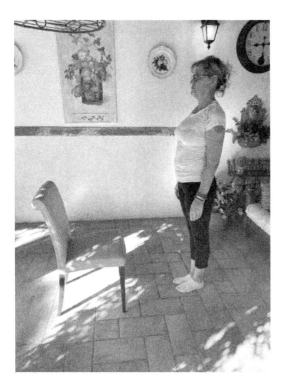 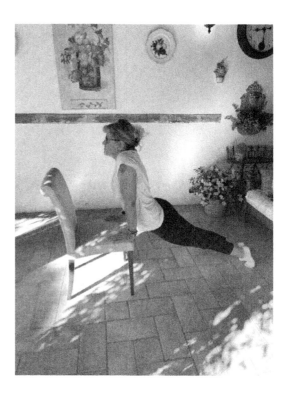

Instructions:

1. Position yourself around three to five feet in front of the chair.

2. Lean forward and rest your hands on the seat in front of you. You should place your hands on the ledges of the seat. Position your body so that it is facing backward at an angle of approximately 45 degrees from the ground. At this time, you ought to be rising on your toes and experiencing a mild stretch in the calf muscles, hip flexors, and hamstrings of your body.

3. Take a long, deep breath in and steadily elevate your chest as you bring your torso into a backbend position. As you bend backward, you ought to experience a stretch in the arms and shoulders of your upper body.

4. If you are at all comfortable doing so, you should tilt your head back and look upward. Maintain this position for a couple of breaths. Make an effort to synchronize your breathing with the stretching you are doing.

5. Take a deep breath in and slowly release your body from the stretch. Then, return to a position where you may relax. If you feel like you have the stamina for it, you can perform this action once more or for a longer period of time.

Seated Shoulder Stretch or Triceps Shoulder Pose

The Seated Shoulder Stretch or Triceps Shoulder Pose is a great yoga exercise that can be adapted for chair yoga to improve upper body mobility and strength. This pose primarily targets the shoulders, triceps, and upper back.

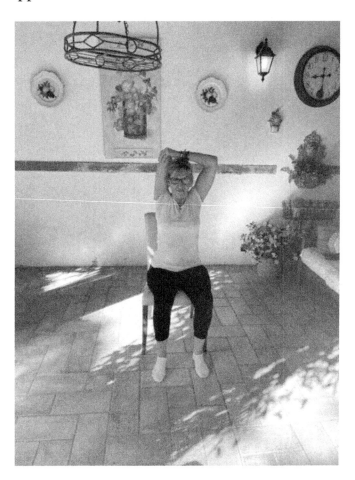

Instructions:

1. Stretch your right hand upward towards the ceiling while seated with your spine in an upright position, legs slightly apart, and feet flat on the floor.

2. Bend your outstretched right hand at the elbow and touch the center of your back. Your shoulder joint should not bend – only your forearm and hand.

3. Take your left hand and place it on your right elbow, and gently press the right elbow gently downwards. This action helps you gain as much stretch on your right shoulder as possible.

4. Hold this stretched position for about 30 seconds.

5. Switch hands and repeat the process with your left hand outstretched this time. Attempt to conduct 3-5 sets of 10 repetitions on each hand.

Reverse Warrior Pose

The Reverse Warrior Pose is a common yoga pose that focuses on stretching and strengthening the upper body, particularly the arms, shoulders, and chest. It's typically done in a standing position, but for chair yoga, we'll need to adapt it.

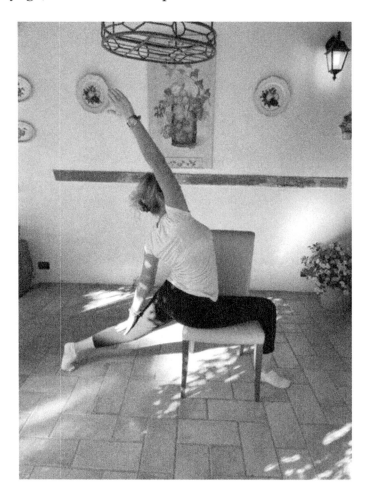

Instructions:

1. Face left as you sit on the chair sideways.

2. Place your right foot on the floor in a flat position and fold your right leg over the seat of the chair. Bring the left leg into a straight position and place the sole of the left foot on the ground so that it is nearly perpendicular to the seat of the chair.

3. Extend your arms out in front of you and bring your right arm forward while simultaneously bringing your left arm behind you.

4. Allow the left arm to come down to the left leg, and then lift the right arm up to the ceiling while keeping the arm straight and ensuring that the hips continue to face forward throughout the entire movement.

5. While maintaining this position, take anywhere from five to eight breaths before transferring to the other side.

6. Repeat five times on each side.

Seated Chest Stretch

A seated chest stretch chair yoga routine can be an excellent way to improve upper body mobility and strength while promoting relaxation and flexibility. This regimen is particularly well-suited for individuals who have extended periods of desk-based sitting or experience restricted mobility.

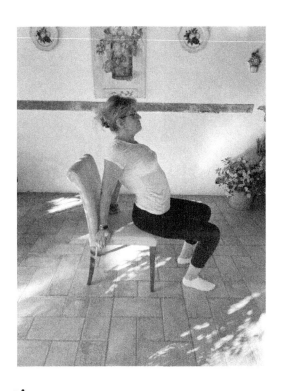 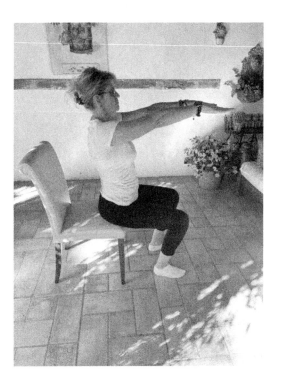

Instructions:

1. Sit up straight and put your feet flat on the floor.

2. Gently lean back and stretch your arms behind you.

3. Hold for about 3 seconds, and then go back to where you started, with your arms out in front of you.

4. Repeat 10 times and rest for 30 seconds before repeating 3 more sets of 10 reps each time.

Seated One-Sided Arm Lifts

Seated one-sided arm lifts are a great chair yoga exercise for improving upper body mobility and strength. This exercise can be especially beneficial for individuals with limited mobility or those who need to perform seated exercises due to physical limitations.

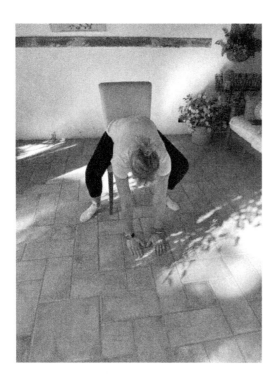 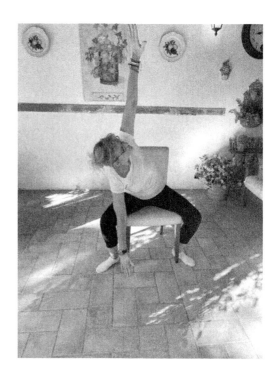

Instructions:

1. Start by sitting down in a nice and comfortable place.

2. Gradually bend into the forward bend position, then take a deep breath.

3. With your hands on the floor, slowly engage your chest and twist to your left as you exhale.

4. Slowly lift your left arm as much as possible, then look up at your arm.

5. Remain in that position for about 20 seconds as you maintain your breathing.

6. Go back to your original position and repeat the same procedure with your right side.

Chapter 7:

Chair Yoga Exercises for People in Post-Surgery Rehab or With Disabilities

Chair yoga exercises hold profound significance for seniors who are in post-surgery rehabilitation or living with disabilities. These gentle and adaptable practices offer a lifeline to individuals facing physical challenges, helping them regain strength, mobility, and overall well-being.

For those in post-surgery rehab, chair yoga provides a safe and effective way to rebuild muscles and flexibility without putting undue strain on the healing body. These exercises promote a gradual return to physical activity, fostering a sense of accomplishment and aiding in the recovery process. Additionally, chair yoga enhances circulation, which is vital for healing, while reducing the risk of post-operative complications such as blood clots.

For seniors with disabilities, chair yoga offers newfound freedom and empowerment. It lets individuals to engage in physical activity regardless of their mobility limitations. The seated and supported poses, combined with controlled breathing, contribute to enhanced balance and coordination. Moreover, chair yoga fosters a sense of community and inclusion, as individuals of varying abilities can participate together, reducing feelings of isolation and boosting mental well-being.

Seated Leg Swings

Seated leg swings chair yoga exercises can be beneficial for people in post-surgery rehab or those with disabilities. Engaging in these exercises can aid in enhancing flexibility, mobility, and strength, all while receiving the benefits of added support and stability.

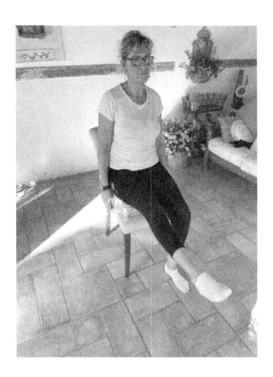 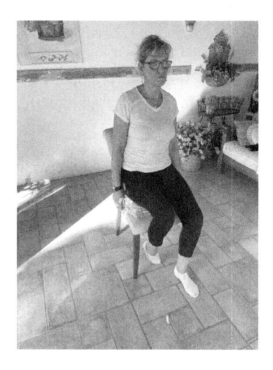

Instructions:

1. Place your feet firmly on the floor and sit on the outside edge of the chair.

2. Hold onto the chair for support.

3. Swing one leg forward and backward gently after placing a small pillow under the thigh, so that the foot doesn't rest on the floor.

4. Repeat on the other side.

5. Perform 10-15 swings on each leg to enhance leg mobility.

Seated Wrist and Hand Exercises

Seated wrist and hand exercises, as well as chair yoga exercises, can be beneficial for individuals in post-surgery rehab or those with disabilities. These exercises can help improve mobility, strength, and flexibility while being gentle on the body.

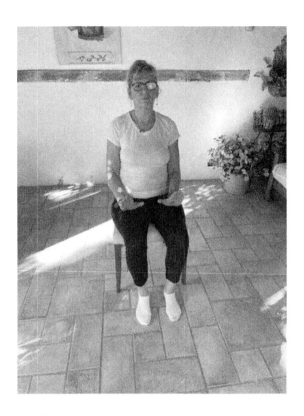 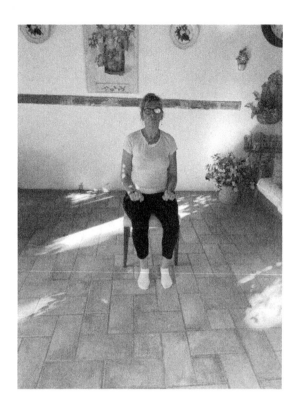

Instructions:

1. Sit with your palms facing down on your thighs.

2. Inhale, lift your fingers toward the ceiling.

3. Exhale, curl your fingers into a fist.

4. Repeat this motion for 10-15 rounds to increase wrist and hand mobility.

Seated Neck Stretches

Seated neck stretches and chair yoga exercises can be incredibly beneficial for people in post-surgery rehab or those with disabilities. These light motions can assist in the reduction of muscle tension, improvement of flexibility, and promotion of relaxation.

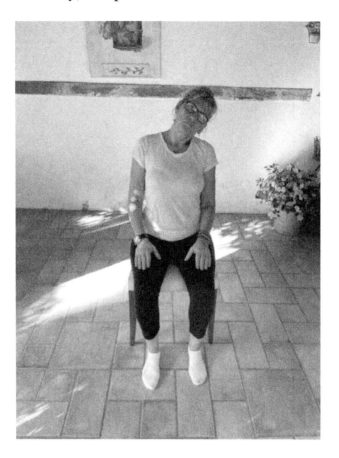

Instructions:

1. Sit upright, ensuring your feet are firmly planted on the ground.

2. Slowly tilt your left ear in the direction of your left shoulder, gently.

3. Hold for a few breaths, then switch sides.

4. Repeat 2-3 times on each side to relieve neck tension.

Seated Bicep Curls

Seated bicep curls are a great way to build strength and improve mobility in the arms for people in post-surgery rehab or with disabilities, especially when performed as part of chair yoga exercises.

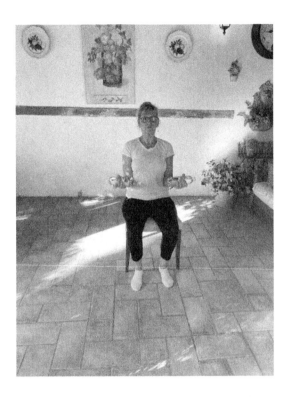 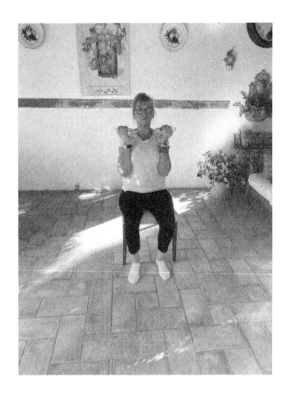

Instructions:

1. Sit with your feet flat on the floor, holding a light weight or water bottle in each hand.

2. Inhale, bend your elbows, and bring the weights toward your shoulders.

3. Exhale, lower the weights.

4. Repeat for 10-15 repetitions to build arm strength.

Seated Heel Raises

Seated heel raises are a gentle chair yoga exercise that can be beneficial for people in post-surgery rehab or those with disabilities. This exercise helps improve ankle strength and flexibility, and it can also aid in improving circulation in the lower legs.

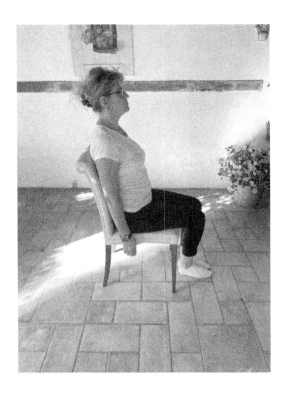 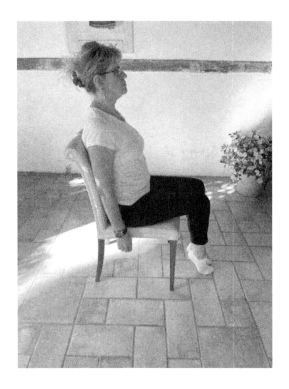

Instructions:

1. Seated position with both feet flat on the floor.

2. Lift both heels off the ground, flexing your calves.

3. Hold for a few breaths and then lower your heels.

4. Repeat 10-15 times to strengthen your calf muscles.

Seated Pigeon Pose

Seated Pigeon Pose is a great chair yoga exercise for individuals in post-surgery rehab or with disabilities because it can help improve flexibility, reduce stiffness, and increase circulation without putting too much strain on the body.

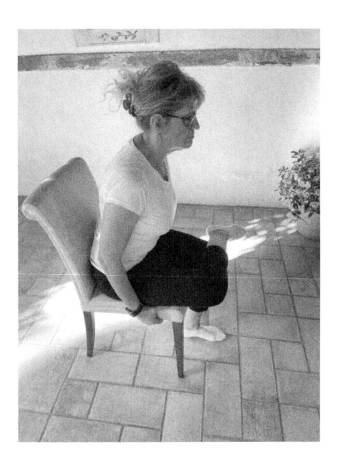

Instructions:

1. While maintaining a stationary position in a chair, open your right hip just a little to the side, lift your right leg, and position your right ankle just above your left knee on your left thigh.

2. Keep flexing your right foot (this will help to engage the muscles that surround your right knee, which will in turn support it).

3. As the right knee comes closer to the ground, slowly sense the hip on the right side release as you keep the spine in a straight position.

Seated Tricep Dips

Seated tricep dips can be adapted for chair yoga exercises suitable for people in post-surgery rehab or with disabilities. These exercises can help improve arm strength and flexibility while seated comfortably in a chair.

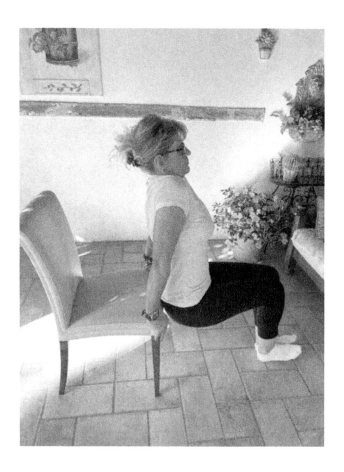

Instructions:

1. Position yourself on the front edge of the chair with your hands resting on the edge of the seat.

2. Walk your feet forward, keeping them flat on the floor.

3. Inhale, bend your elbows, and lower your hips towards the floor.

4. Exhale, push back up.

5. Repeat 10-15 times to work on triceps strength.

Seated Pelvic Tilts

Seated pelvic tilts are gentle chair yoga exercises that can be particularly beneficial for people in post-surgery rehab or with disabilities. Engaging in these exercises can contribute to enhancing flexibility, mobility, and blood circulation, all while fostering a sense of relaxation.

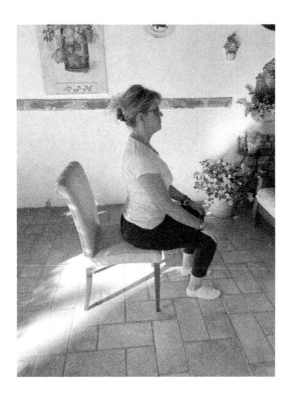 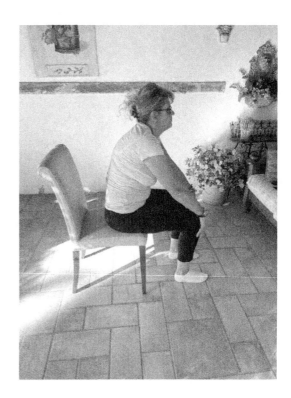

Instructions:

1. Sit upright, ensuring your feet are firmly planted on the ground.

2. Inhale, arch your lower back slightly, sticking your chest out.

3. Exhale, round your lower back, tucking your pelvis under.

4. Repeat this gentle tilting motion to improve pelvic mobility.

Seated Relaxation with Visualization

Seated Relaxation with Visualization is a simple chair yoga pose that combines gentle movements with guided imagery to promote relaxation and reduce stress.

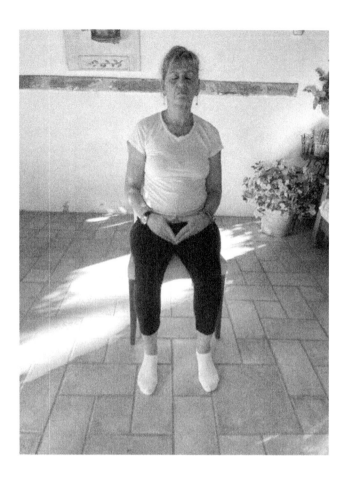

Instructions:

1. Sit back in the chair with your eyes closed.

2. Take several deep breaths and imagine a peaceful, calming place.

3. Spend a few minutes in this relaxed state, visualizing your serene environment.

Seated Quad Stretch

Seated quad stretches can be beneficial for individuals in post-surgery rehab or those with disabilities as they allow for gentle stretching and strengthening of the quadriceps muscles while providing stability and support.

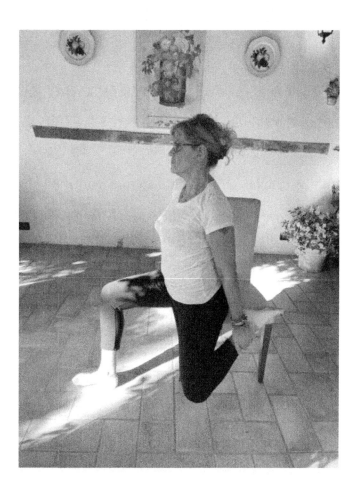

Instructions:

1. Take a seat in the corner of the chair with both feet flat on the floor.

2. Grasp your left ankle and gently draw it towards your buttocks.

3. Hold for a few breaths, then switch legs.

4. This stretch targets the quadriceps.

Chapter 8:

14 Simple Chair Yoga Pose to Choose for Your 10 Minutes Daily Routine

Chair yoga offers seniors a gentle yet effective means of staying physically active. With age, mobility can become more challenging. However, these thoughtfully selected poses assist in enhancing balance, flexibility, and strength, consequently reducing the risk of falls and injuries.

Mental well-being is equally crucial. Daily chair yoga routines promote relaxation, stress reduction, and mental clarity. The slow, mindful movements, combined with controlled breathing, create a sense of calm and presence, alleviating anxiety and enhancing mental focus.

Chair yoga is an inclusive discipline that can be customized to accommodate diverse fitness levels and physical constraints, rendering it accessible to a broad spectrum of seniors. This inclusiveness cultivates a feeling of belonging and empowerment, bolstering self-esteem and the overall quality of life.

Consistency is key, and a brief daily routine ensures that seniors reap the cumulative benefits of chair yoga. These 14 simple poses provide a well-rounded practice, targeting different muscle groups and aspects of well-being, making it a time-efficient yet comprehensive addition to their daily lives.

Chair Lunge Pose

This chair yoga exercise works by flexing your hips and groin area. It also tones and stretches your legs, especially your thighs, and boosts the strength of your waist, knees, and ankles. This exercise also stretches your chest by lengthening your spine and stimulates the organs found around the abdominal area.

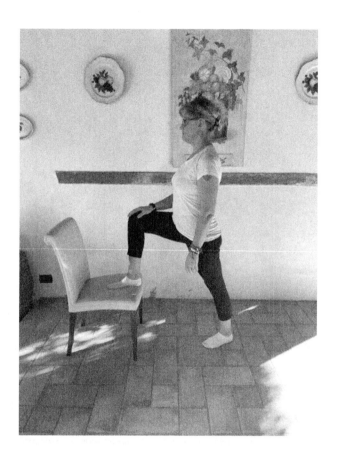

Instructions:

1. Once again, stand at arms-length in front of your chair, lift your right leg and place it onto the chair's sitting space.

2. If you prefer some balance support, turn the chair so that the backrest is on your right or left side – depending on which leg you are working on. All your body weight will transfer to the leg on the ground—in this case, the left leg.

3. Now slowly lean forward towards your right leg elevated on the seat. You should feel some stretch in the front of your right hip and calf area.

4. Ensure your knee aligns with your ankle and is not behind or in front of it. Next, turn to your left leg and stretch it as well. You can perform five repetitions for each leg.

Seated Child's Pose (Balasana)

Seated Child's Pose, adapted for chair yoga, is a restorative and gentle stretch that can help seniors improve their posture and find relief from tension in the lower back. It's an excellent way to relax and rejuvenate during your chair yoga practice.

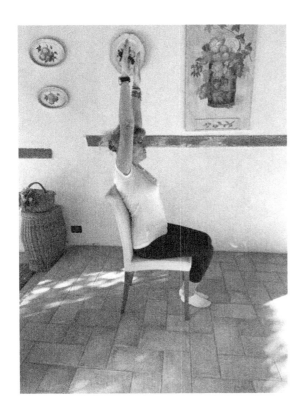 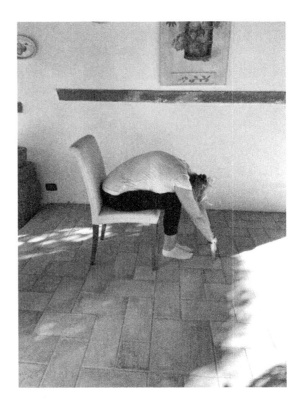

Instructions:

1. Sit upright, ensuring your feet are firmly planted on the ground.

2. Inhale, raise your arms overhead.

3. Exhale, bend forward at your hips, reaching your hands toward the floor.

4. Hold for 20-30 secs, breathing deeply.

Half-Moon Pose

Unlike the other chair yoga poses, this one requires you to stand on your feet; however, you'll still rely on the chair for support. This workout routine is great for strengthening many muscles in your body, like the chest, hamstrings, upper back and shoulders, core and arm muscles. The pose is also great for improving circulation and flexibility.

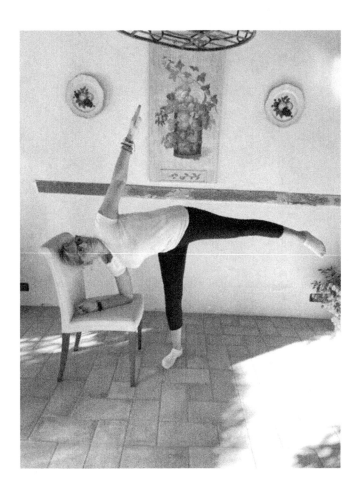

Instructions:

1. Start by standing straight in front of the seat.

2. Inhale, then slowly lower your body until you touch the seat with your hands. Go lower again until you place your forearm on the seat.

3. Use your right hand for support, then raise your left hand.

4. Slowly lift your left leg until it is perpendicular to your body. Ensure you're balanced, with your right forearm is offering enough support.

5. Remain in that position for about 20 seconds before returning to your original position.

6. Repeat the same procedure with your left side.

Thread the Needle

Thread the Needle is a popular yoga pose that can be adapted for chair yoga to improve lower body mobility and strength. Chair yoga serves as an excellent choice for individuals with restricted mobility or those who favor a seated practice.

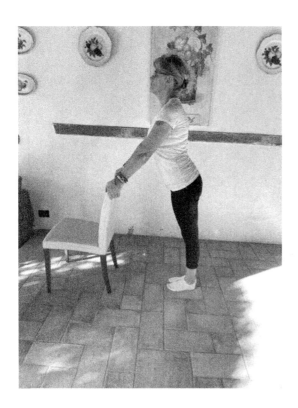 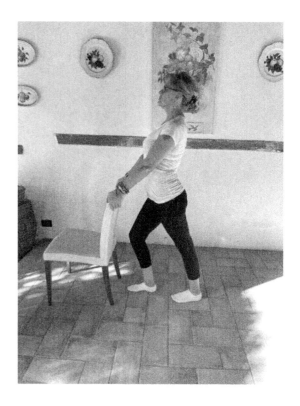

Instructions:

1. Whilst standing behind the chair, place your hands on the back of the chair so that your fingers are approximately shoulder-width apart.

2. Place your hands on the outside of the chair and take a step back with your feet.

3. Put your right foot forward and take a step forward.

4. Once you shift your weight to the rear, you ought to feel a sense of comfort on the right side of your torso.

5. While you are pulling the right hand carefully make sure to keep your back straight and your abdominal muscles tight.

6. Upon maintaining the stance for a moment, repeat the exercise on the other side.

Seated Butterfly Stretch Variation

The Seated Butterfly Stretch is a simple chair yoga pose that can help improve flexibility & release tension in the hips and groin area. This variation is ideal for those who have difficulty sitting on the floor or need extra support.

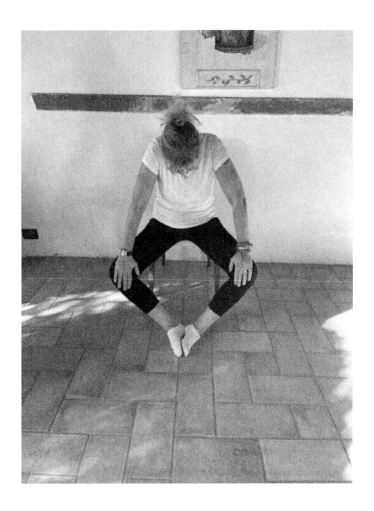

Instructions:

1. Sit upright, ensuring your feet are firmly planted on the ground.

2. Bring the soles of your feet together, letting your knees drop out to the sides.

3. Gently press your knees toward the floor.

4. Inhale, lift your chest.

5. Exhale, hinge at your hips, then lean forward slightly.

6. Hold for a few breaths.

Seated Eagle Pose

This posture is beneficial for enhancing focus and concentration, as well as shoulder movement, upper back flexibility, and stretching. In addition, it stretches and loosens the upper back. Because the seated eagle stance is not particularly strenuous, even elderly people are able to perform it. It is additionally suggested for those who suffer from pain in the neck or upper back. Additionally, it is beneficial for cases of arthritis that affect the joints of the hands, especially the wrists, elbows, and fingers.

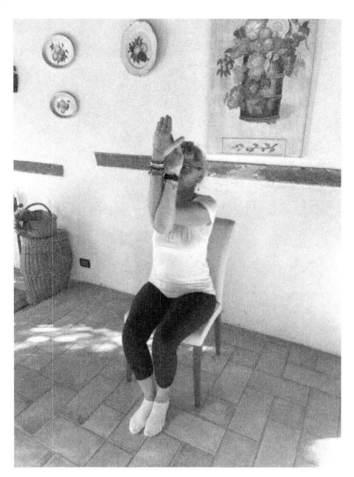

Instructions:

1. While sitting in the chair, maintain an upright posture with both feet planted firmly on the floor in a position where they are parallel to one another and separated by a distance equal to the width of your hips.

2. Extend both of your arms to the side of your body.

3. Put them towards your body, bend your elbows, and cross your upper arms so that your right arm is on top of your left arm.

4. Bring your palms together in front of your face and conceal your forearms over one another so that they meet in the middle.

5. Maintain a position in which your upper arms are parallel to your thighs.

6. Remain in this position for six to eight full breaths.

7. Remove your arms from the cross position, and then repeat moves 2 through 6 on the other side of your body.

Sage Marichi Pose

This is an intense pose engaging the gluteal muscles and abdominal muscles, as well as the chest, shoulders, arms, and hands. It stretches the right and left leg muscles similarly to how the psoas or quadriceps and hip flexor muscles are stretched.

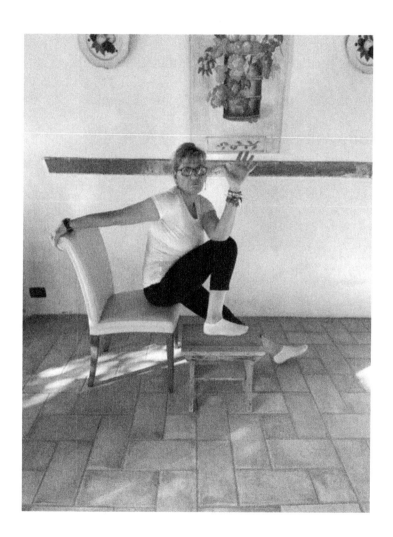

Instructions:

1. Place two blocks stacked near the right side of the chair.

2. Sit on the chair's edge, relax for 3-4 breaths, stretching your back.

3. Spread legs in front and place your right foot on blocks.

4. Stretch left leg forward, heel touching floor, toes flexed, feel calf stretch.

5. Keep right foot on blocks, bend knees and hips.

6. Sit upright, twist upper body right, holding chair's back with right hand.

7. Left arm to right thigh, left elbow outside right thigh. Press elbow on knee, feel stretch in upper outer thigh and abs.

8. Twist spine further, engaging back, shoulders, chest, and stomach.

9. Start slow breathing, deepen twist with each exhale.

10. Stay for 3-4 breaths, push feet to blocks, elbows to knee, maintain alignment.

11. Engage back, chest, abs, and glutes while holding.

12. Release elbow, relax head, let go of hands and legs to sit up.

13. After deep breathing, repeat, twist left, left foot on blocks.

14. Hold for 3-4 breaths, release, relax.

Camel Pose

There are several variations of this pose, but the one in focus here is the camel chair pose. This is a very simple but effective yoga pose that is great for improving flexibility and circulation in your body.

The camel pose with chair pose is great for strengthening a wide range of muscles in the body, like the back, hips, arms, and core muscles. It is the less strenuous form of the normal camel pose that requires you to go all the way down to your feet.

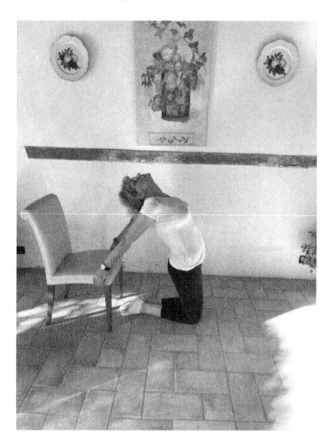

Instructions:

1. Begin by standing close to a chair but with your back facing it. Make sure to stand a few inches from the chair to give enough room to your legs once you kneel.

2. Carefully kneel and bring your arms backward such that they can hold the seat behind you.

3. Now slowly lean back as much as you can until you face upwards. Make sure to keep your feet together and in between the chair.

4. Remain in that position for about 20 seconds before returning to your original position. Repeat this process for ten reps while making sure you bend backward as much as possible.

Seated Cow Face Arms

The "Seated Cow Face Arms" is a yoga pose that primarily focuses on stretching the shoulders and upper back. It's a great option for a simple chair yoga routine.

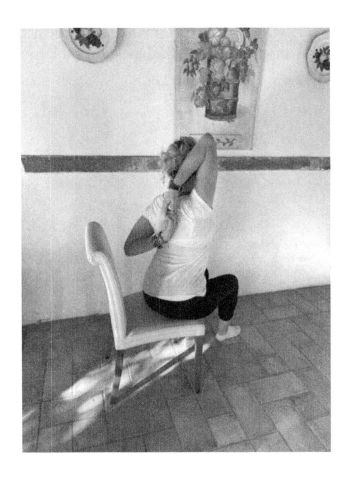

Instructions:

1. Sit up straight.

2. Inhale, extend your right arm up.

3. Exhale, bend your right elbow and reach your hand down your back.

4. Inhale, extend your left arm out to the side.

5. Exhale, bend your left elbow then reach your hand up your back.

6. If possible, clasp your hands behind your back.

7. Hold for a few breaths.

Upward Plank Pose

The Upward Plank Pose, also known as Purvottanasana in yoga, is a challenging pose that offers numerous benefits, including strengthening the arms, wrists, and legs, improving posture, and stretching the front of the body.

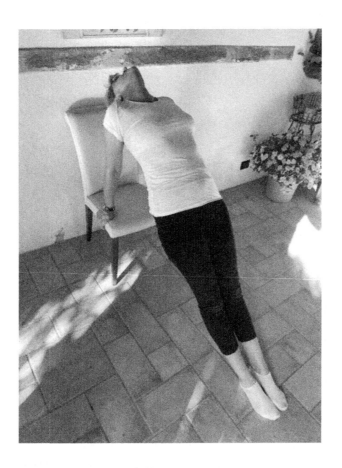

Instructions:

1. Sit upright with your legs stretched straight before you.

2. Now place your hands beside your hips before slowly taking them about an inch behind your back with your elbows slightly bent.

3. Make sure your hands are strong enough to hold your weight before lifting your torso slowly from the chair all the way up as much as possible.

4. Remain in that position for about 20 seconds before returning to your original position. Repeat this process about 20 times until you feel your core and leg muscles have become loose enough.

Seated Corpse Pose

This full-body stretch is often the victim of neglect despite the numerous benefits to your body and mind. The pose allows your body to let go, feel heavy and do nothing, quieting down previously active systems at its own pace. You will need some leg support for this pose in the form of a pillow or cushion.

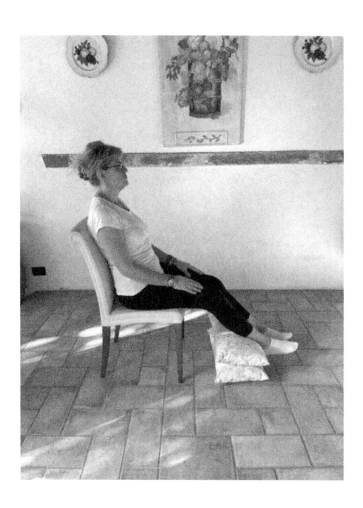

Instructions:

1. Sit with your feet stretched out straight, toes pointing up, and your back reclined at an angle to rest on your chair's rest.

2. Place a pillow or cushion underneath your feet to cushion them from the floor's hardness and cold and elevate them slightly for improved blood circulation.

3. Let your hands dangle towards the floor or rest them on your lap. Close your eyes, take deep breaths to relax, and allow your body to normalize your breathing pattern at its natural pace.

4. Remain in repose while listening to the sensations in your body, and set your thoughts free to wander until you feel refreshed, relaxed, and rejuvenated.

Seated Bridge Pose Variation

The Seated Bridge Pose variation in Chair Yoga is a gentle and accessible yoga pose that can help improve posture, strengthen the back and core, and increase flexibility.

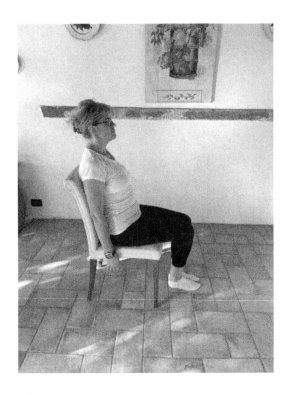 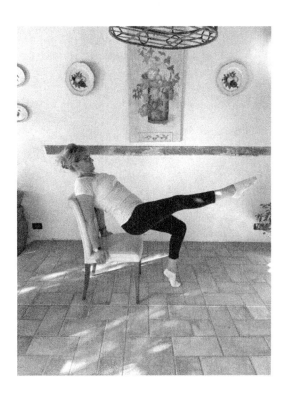

Instructions:

1. Sit with your feet flat on the floor and hands resting on the chair's sides.

2. Inhale, lift your hips, and engage your glutes.

3. Extend one leg straight in front of you.

4. Hold for a few breaths, then switch legs.

Seated Boat Pose with Twist

Seated Boat Pose with Twist is a variation of the traditional Boat Pose (Navasana) that can be adapted for chair yoga. It's a great pose for strengthening the core muscles and improving balance.

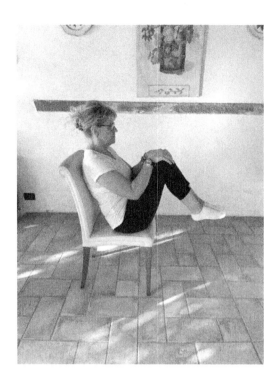 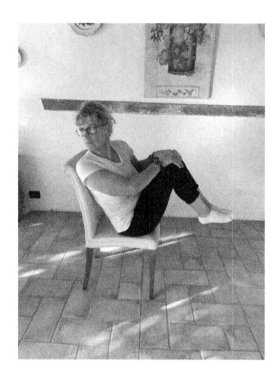

Instructions:

1. Position yourself at the chair's edge, making sure your feet are resting flat on the floor.

2. Inhale, lift your feet off the ground.

3. Exhale, engage your core, and twist your torso to the right.

4. Hold for a few breaths, then switch sides.

Seated Child's Pose Variation

The Seated Child's Pose Variation is a simple Chair Yoga pose that can help promote relaxation and flexibility, even if you have limited mobility. This variation adapts the traditional Child's Pose to make it accessible while sitting in a chair.

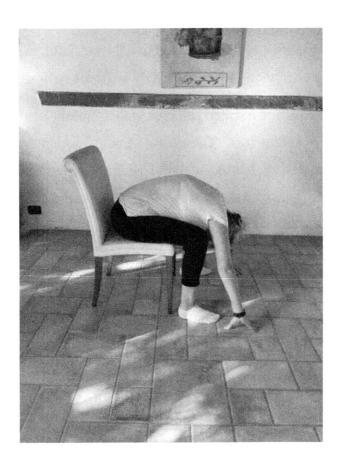

Instructions:

1. Maintain a seated position with both feet resting flat on the floor.

2. Spread your knees apart then bring your chest towards your thighs.

3. Extend your arms forward until your hands touch the floor.

4. Hold for a few breaths, then release.

Chapter 9:

Bonus: 15 Chair Exercises for Weight Loss

For older adults, traditional vigorous workouts may pose challenges, making chair exercises a valuable alternative. These exercises are designed to cater to reduced mobility and varying fitness levels, allowing seniors to engage in physical activity without straining their bodies.

Chair exercises provide an avenue to burn calories, boost metabolism, and enhance muscle tone, all of which contribute to weight loss. These low-impact movements, such as seated leg lifts, seated marches, and seated twists, enable seniors to engage major muscle groups without putting undue stress on joints. By incorporating resistance bands or light hand weights, seniors can further intensify their workouts while remaining seated.

Consistency in chair exercises supports gradual weight loss and maintenance, and it can lead to improved cardiovascular health, better circulation, and enhanced flexibility. Additionally, these exercises positively impact mental well-being, helping seniors manage stress and elevate their mood.

Seated Triangle Pose

The Triangle pose can help increase stability, open the hips and shoulders, and lengthen the spine. However, it can be a complicated movement for those with limited flexibility, so it may take time to become proficient. The important thing is to listen to your body and not stretch further than your body can. Also, during this exercise, care should be taken not to overbalance as you will be leaning forward in the chair.

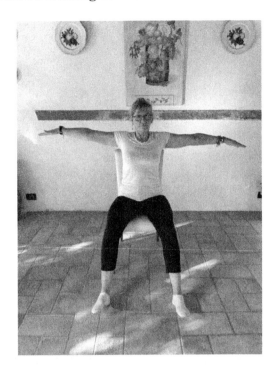 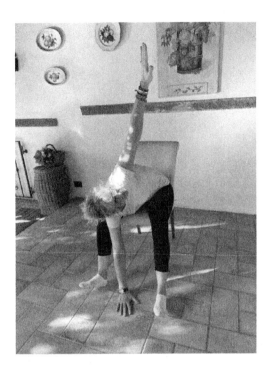

Instructions:

1. Find a comfortable sitting position in a chair, spreading your legs wide in front of you and keeping them flat on the floor.

2. As you breathe in, extend your arms out to the sides at shoulder height.

3. Exhale and twist your body so that your right-hand points towards the floor. Your left hand should be pointing towards the ceiling. Touch the floor with your right hand if you can but extend your left hand up as far as you can. Turn your neck so that you are looking up at the ceiling.

4. Hold this pose for 30 secs, if you can.

5. On an inhale, bring your body back to the starting position with your arms parallel to the floor.

6. Repeat this movement on the other side.

7. Repeat the entire exercise three times on each side.

Seated Warrior III with Twist

Seated Warrior III with Twist Chair Exercise is a modified version of the yoga pose Warrior III that can be done while seated in a chair. This exercise can help improve balance, strengthen your core muscles, and increase flexibility. While it may not be as intense as some other exercises for weight loss, it can still contribute to your overall fitness routine.

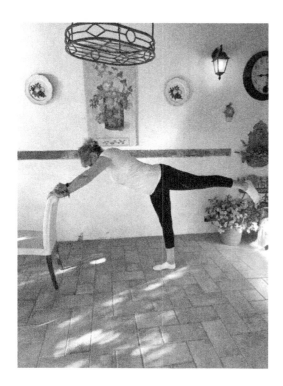 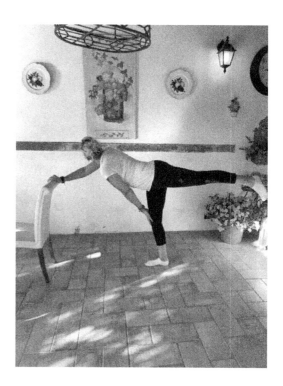

Instructions:

1. Begin by standing in the back of your chair.

2. Extend one leg straight to the back.

3. Inhale, extend your arms forward.

4. Exhale, twist your torso to the right, bringing your left hand to your right knee.

5. Hold for a few breaths, then switch sides.

Seated Finger-to-Toe Stretch

Seated finger-to-toe stretch chair exercises can be a great addition to your weight loss routine, especially if you have limited mobility or find it difficult to engage in more vigorous activities. These stretches can help improve flexibility, circulation, and overall mobility. However, it's essential to remember that while stretching exercises can be beneficial, weight loss primarily relies on a combination of a balanced diet and regular physical activity, which includes cardiovascular exercises and strength training.

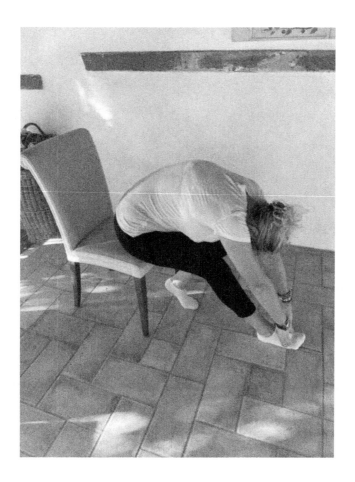

Instructions:

1. Sit with your feet flat on the floor.

2. Inhale, reach forward and try to touch your toes.

3. Exhale, relax and return to a seated position.

4. Repeat this stretch for 10-15 rounds to enhance flexibility.

Seated Modified Fish Pose

Seated Modified Fish Pose Chair Exercise is a variation of the traditional yoga pose that can be adapted for individuals with mobility limitations or those who prefer to exercise while sitting in a chair. It can be a part of a broader exercise routine that includes cardiovascular exercises and a balanced diet for effective weight management.

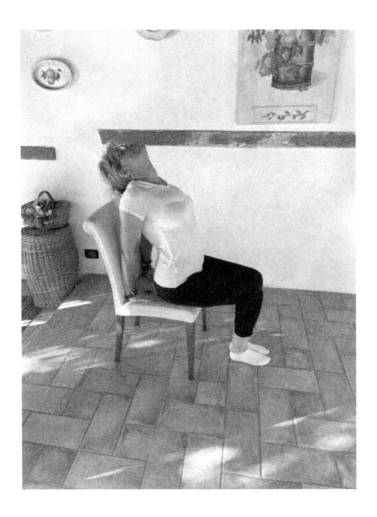

Instructions:

1. Take a seat in the chair, ensuring your feet are flat on the floor.

2. Inhale deeply as you raise your chest and gently arch your back.

3. Hold for a few breaths.

4. Exhale and release.

Seated Wide-Legged Forward Fold

Seated wide-legged forward fold chair exercises can be a great addition to your weight loss routine, especially if you have mobility issues or are looking for low-impact options. These exercises can help you strengthen your core, improve flexibility, and burn calories.

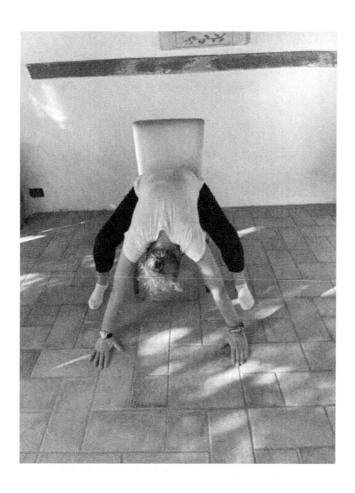

Instructions:

1. Sit forward in the chair with your feet wider than hip-width apart.

2. Inhale, lengthen your spine.

3. Exhale, hinge at your hips, and reach your hands towards the floor.

4. Hold for a gentle stretch.

Seated Figure Stretch

Seated figure stretch chair exercises can be a great way to incorporate physical activity into your routine if you have mobility issues or prefer seated workouts. These exercises can help improve your flexibility, strengthen your muscles, and boost your metabolism when combined with a healthy diet & overall active lifestyle.

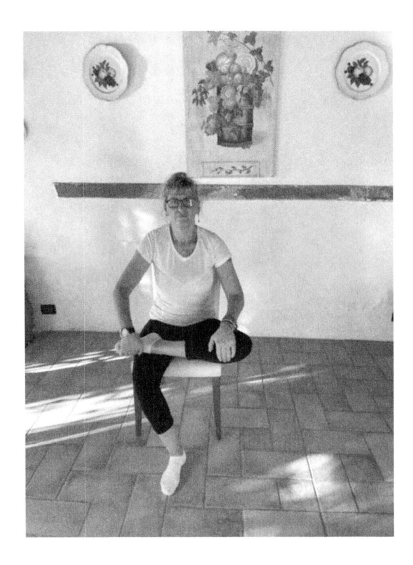

Instructions:

1. Be seated, ensuring that your feet are resting flat on the floor.

2. Proceed by crossing your left ankle over your right knee.

3. Gently press down on your left knee.

4. Hold for a few breaths, then switch sides.

Seated Reverse Warrior

Seated reverse warrior chair exercises can be an effective way to engage your core, strengthen your lower body, and promote weight loss. These exercises are suitable for people with limited mobility or those who prefer seated workouts.

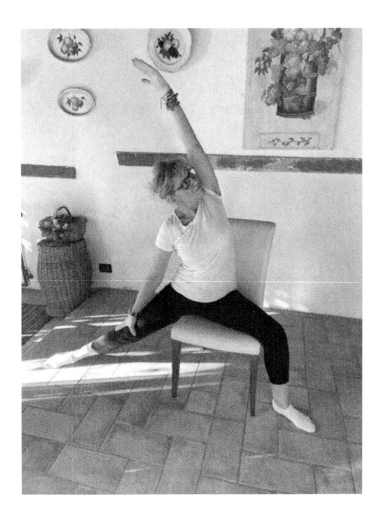

Instructions:

1. Sit with your feet flat on the floor.

2. Extend your right leg straight to the side.

3. Inhale, reach your left arm overhead.

4. Exhale, slide your right hand down your extended leg.

5. Hold for a few breaths, then switch sides.

Seated Abdominal Twists

Seated abdominal twists are a great chair exercise for engaging your core muscles and potentially aiding in weight loss when combined with a balanced diet and overall fitness routine. These exercises can help strengthen your obliques and improve your posture.

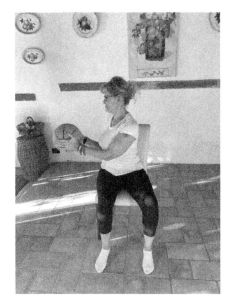 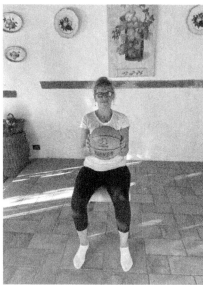 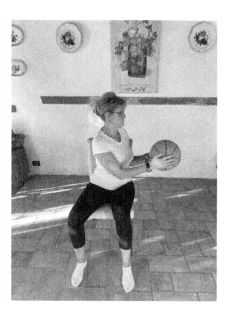

Instructions:

1. Sit upright, ensuring your feet are firmly planted on the ground.

2. Hold a ball or pillow in both hands.

3. Inhale and twist your torso to the right, bringing the ball or pillow to your right hip.

4. Exhale, return to the center.

5. Repeat on the left side.

6. Perform 10-15 twists on each side to engage your core.

Seated Supported Boat Pose

Seated Supported Boat Pose is a modified version of the traditional Boat Pose (Navasana) from yoga, which can be performed in a chair.

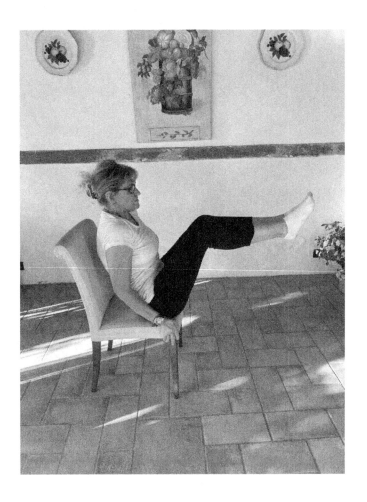

Instructions:

1. Position yourself on the front edge of the chair, making sure your feet are resting flat on the floor.

2. Hold the sides of the chair for support.

3. Inhale, lift your feet off the ground.

4. Exhale, engage your core, and hold.

5. Hold for a few breaths.

Seated Supine Twist

The Seated Supine Twist is a gentle chair yoga pose that can help stretch and release tension in the spine and improve flexibility. It's a modification of the traditional Supine Twist, adapted for those who may have difficulty getting down to the floor.

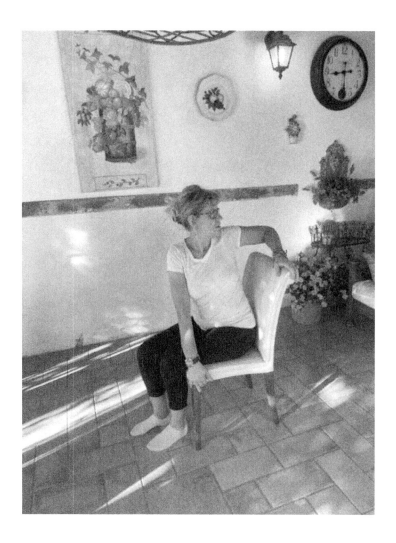

Instructions:

1. Sit towards the edge of your chair.

2. Inhale, lengthen your spine.

3. Exhale, twist to the left and hold the backrest of the chair.

4. Hold for a few breaths, then switch sides.

Seated Shoulder Blade Squeeze

Seated shoulder blade squeeze exercises can be a helpful addition to your weight loss routine, especially if you spend a lot of time sitting at a desk or in front of a computer. These exercises can improve posture and help activate the muscles in your upper back, which can aid in burning calories and supporting your overall weight loss goals.

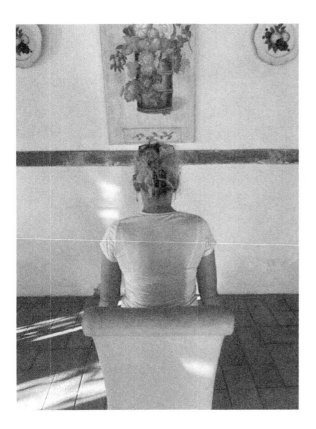 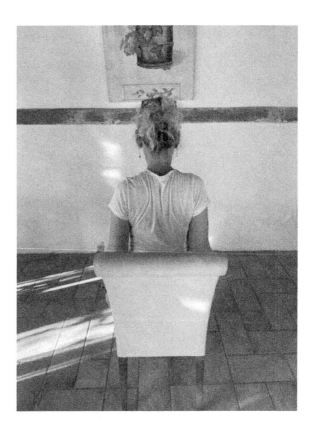

Instructions:

1. Sit upright, ensuring your feet are firmly planted on the ground.

2. Inhale, squeeze your shoulder blades together.

3. Exhale, release.

4. Repeat for 10-15 rounds to improve posture and relieve tension in the upper back.

Seated Camel Pose with Chair Support

Seated Camel Pose with chair support is a yoga pose that can be incorporated into a weight loss routine to help improve flexibility, strengthen your core, and increase overall body awareness. While it may not be a high-intensity exercise for weight loss on its own, it can complement a balanced fitness program.

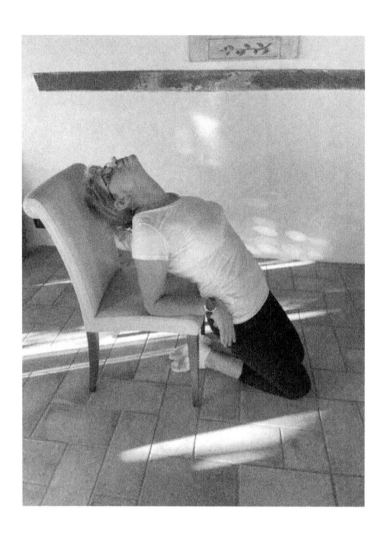

Instructions:

1. Start by standing next to a chair, but with your back facing it. Be sure to stand a few inches from the chair to give your legs room when you kneel.

2. Kneel carefully and bring your arms back so that your elbows rest on the seat behind you.

3. At this point, slowly lean back as far as you can until your face is facing upward. Be sure to keep your feet together and in the center of the chair.

4. Stay in this position for about 20 seconds before returning to the starting position. Repeat this process ten times, making sure to lean back as far as possible.

Dancer's Pose

The chest, shoulders, and fronts of the thighs are all given more space when the dancer is in this position. The dancer's position is a jubilant posture that is going to make you pleased each and every time you execute it. This position is useful for a number of reasons, including the strengthening of the legs and the core in addition to the improvement of balance.

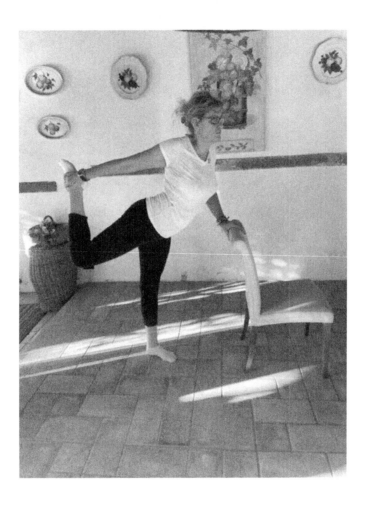

Instructions:

1. Start by positioning yourself to the left of the chairs back as you stand there. Put your right hand behind your back and put your left hand on the back of the chair. Then, use your right hand to turn around and grab the top of your right foot.

2. Extend your right leg behind you as you bring your chest forward and open out all of your front torso while bending your right knee behind you.

3. Exhale slowly and hold your breath for five to eight seconds. Repeat the exercise with the other leg.

Modified Planks

Seated modified planks can be an effective exercise to incorporate into your weight loss routine. Planks are a great way to engage your core muscles, which can help you build strength and increase your metabolism.

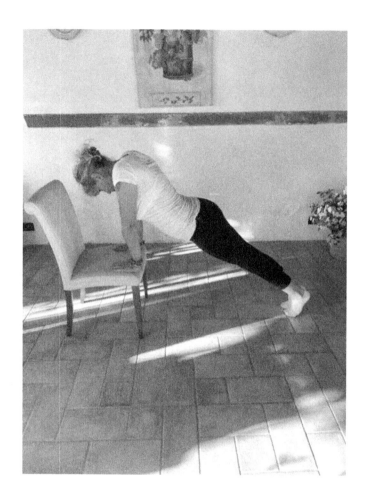

Instructions:

1. Stand straight and face the chair.

2. Hold the chair's sides with both hands. Slightly bend your elbow and move your feet behind till your body is in a diagonal position to the chair.

3. Keep your back straight and your buttocks down. Maintain a straight line from your shoulder to your heel. When a senior feel resistance or stress in their core, this indicates that they are in the appropriate position.

4. Hold this position for thirty seconds (or for as long as is comfortable without causing pain), and then go into a standing or seated position to give yourself a little break.

5. Repeat 2 to 3 times.

Seated Relaxation with Breath Awareness

Seated relaxation with breath awareness chair exercises can be a helpful addition to a weight loss plan. These exercises can help reduce stress, improve mindfulness, and burn a small number of calories. While they won't replace more vigorous forms of exercise, they can be a great option for people who have mobility issues or are looking for gentle ways to incorporate movement into their routine.

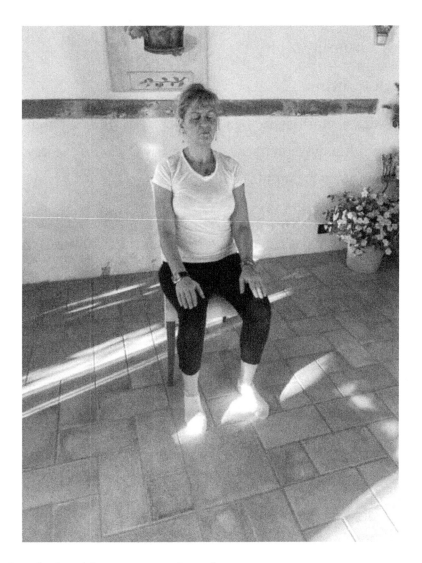

1. Sit back in the chair with your eyes closed.

2. Take several deep breaths and focus on your breath.

3. Pay attention to the expansion and contraction of your chest and the feeling of your breath flowing in and out of your body.

4. Spend a few minutes in this relaxed state, calming your mind and body.

Chapter 10:

Integrating Chair Yoga into Daily Life

Now, let's delve into the practical aspects of incorporating chair yoga into your daily life. Chair yoga isn't just an exercise; it's a holistic practice that enhances physical and mental well-being. By integrating chair yoga into your daily routine, you can experience its transformative effects on your health and overall quality of life.

Morning Chair Yoga Routine:

1. Start your day with a short chair yoga routine. A few minutes of gentle stretching, deep breathing, and mindful movement can set a positive tone for the day. Focus on awakening your body and calming your mind.

2. Incorporate stretches that target areas of tension or stiffness, such as the neck, shoulders, & lower back. These stretches can help alleviate morning stiffness and improve flexibility.

3. Practice deep abdominal breathing to oxygenate your body and boost your energy levels. A few rounds of diaphragmatic breathing can invigorate you for the day ahead.

Chair Yoga at Work:

1. If you have a desk job, use chair yoga to combat the negative effects of prolonged sitting. Incorporate short chair yoga breaks throughout the workday to stretch and re-energize.

2. Simple seated stretches, wrist and ankle rotations, and neck stretches can be done discreetly at your desk. These movements help improve circulation, reduce tension, and enhance concentration.

3. Practice chair yoga during lunch breaks to relieve stress and mental fatigue. A brief mindfulness meditation session or deep breathing exercises can be particularly rejuvenating.

Evening Relaxation Routine:

1. Wind down in the evening with a chair yoga routine designed for relaxation. Focus on gentle stretches and deep breathing to release tension accumulated during the day.

2. Incorporate poses that promote relaxation, such as forward bends, gentle twists, and restorative poses. These poses can prepare your body for restful sleep.

3. Practice mindfulness meditation before bedtime to quiet the mind and promote a sense of inner peace. This can enhance the quality of your sleep.

Chair Yoga for Stress Management:

1. Whenever you encounter stress or tension, turn to chair yoga as a coping mechanism. Deep breathing exercises and relaxation poses can help alleviate stress and calm the nervous system.

2. Develop a "stress toolkit" of chair yoga techniques that you can use in stressful situations. These may include quick relaxation exercises or breathing techniques to regain composure.

3. Consider incorporating chair yoga into your daily routine as a proactive approach to stress management. Regular practice can increase resilience to stressors.

Social Chair Yoga:

1. Share the benefits of chair yoga with friends or family members. Invite them to join you in a chair yoga session, creating a supportive and social experience.

2. Organize chair yoga gatherings or classes within your community or social groups. Chair yoga is accessible to individuals of varying ages and physical capabilities, creating an inclusive practice that can be enjoyed by everyone.

3. Practicing chair yoga with others fosters a sense of connection and well-being, enhancing the social aspect of your daily life.

Adaptation for Special Needs:

1. If you have physical limitations or specific health conditions, work with a qualified chair yoga instructor to adapt poses and techniques to your unique needs.

2. Integrating chair yoga into your daily life may require modifications to accommodate your abilities and limitations. These modifications ensure that chair yoga remains a safe and enjoyable practice.

Chair yoga isn't limited to a studio or gym; it's a practice that can seamlessly weave into your daily life. By integrating chair yoga into your routines, you can experience its profound benefits, from improved physical flexibility to reduced stress and enhanced mindfulness. Embrace chair yoga as a lifelong companion on your journey to holistic well-being.

Chapter 11:

Frequently Asked Questions and Troubleshooting Relaxation and Stress Relief

In the pursuit of relaxation and stress relief, questions often arise. Here are some frequently asked questions (FAQs) and troubleshooting tips to help you navigate your journey to greater tranquility and well-being.

What is the best time to practice relaxation techniques like chair yoga?

Relaxation techniques can be practiced at any time that suits your schedule and preferences. Some people find morning practices invigorating, while others prefer winding down with relaxation techniques in the evening. Experiment with different times to find what works best for you.

I have trouble quieting my mind during relaxation. What can I do?

Mindfulness meditation and deep breathing can help calm a busy mind. If you find it challenging to focus, try guided meditations or soothing music to assist in relaxation. It's normal for thoughts to arise; acknowledge them without judgment and gently redirect your focus to your breath or the meditation.

How long should I practice relaxation techniques each day?

The duration of your practice can vary based on your schedule and needs. Even a few minutes of relaxation techniques can be beneficial. However, aiming for 10 to 20 minutes daily can have a noticeable impact on your stress levels and overall well-being.

I'm having difficulty achieving a deep state of relaxation. What should I do?

Achieving a deep state of relaxation can take time and practice. Be patient with yourself. Explore different relaxation techniques to find what resonates with you. Guided imagery, progressive muscle relaxation, or body scans are techniques that can deepen relaxation.

I sometimes feel more stressed or anxious after relaxation. Is this normal?

Occasionally, you may become more aware of underlying stress or tension during relaxation. This is a sign that your body is beginning to release stored stress. Continue with your practice, and over time, this sensation should diminish as you become more adept at releasing stress.

What should I do if I fall asleep during relaxation exercises?

Falling asleep during relaxation is common, especially if you're fatigued. While relaxation is the goal, if you'd like to remain awake, try practicing in a seated position instead of lying down or experiment with keeping your eyes open during your practice.

I'm experiencing physical discomfort during relaxation exercises. What can I do to alleviate this?

If you're experiencing discomfort, adjust your posture or try using additional props, such as cushions or blankets, for support. Make sure you're not tensing your muscles unnecessarily. The goal is to relax both mentally & physically.

Can relaxation techniques replace medical treatment for stress-related conditions?

While relaxation techniques can provide valuable support alongside medical treatment for stress-related issues, it's important to note that they should not replace professional medical advice and care. If you're dealing with a medical condition or mental health issue, it's advisable to seek guidance from a healthcare provider.

How do I maintain a consistent relaxation practice?

To maintain consistency, schedule relaxation sessions at a specific time each day or incorporate them into your existing routine. Enlist the support of a friend or family member to practice with you or remind you. Tracking your progress in a journal can also motivate you to stick with it.

What if I don't feel immediate relief from stress after practicing relaxation techniques?

Stress relief through relaxation techniques often accumulates gradually. It may take time to notice significant changes in your stress levels. Be patient, and trust that consistent practice will yield positive results in the long run.

Conclusion

Maintaining a Lifelong Chair Yoga Practice

Incorporating chair yoga into your life is not merely an exercise routine; it's a lifelong commitment to holistic well-being. As you've discovered throughout this journey, chair yoga offers a myriad of physical, mental, and emotional benefits that can enrich your quality of life at any age. To maintain a lifelong chair yoga practice, embrace it as an essential part of your daily routine. Whether you're starting your day with gentle stretches, taking short chair yoga breaks at work, or winding down with relaxation poses in the evening, chair yoga becomes a trusted companion on your journey to a healthier and more harmonious existence. Remember, consistency is key, and even small, regular sessions can yield profound results over time. Embrace chair yoga not as an obligation but as an act of self-care and self-love, nurturing your body, mind, and spirit for years to come. With the knowledge and techniques you've acquired, may your chair yoga practice continue to be a source of strength, tranquility, and lifelong well-being.

Celebrating Your Progress and Well-being

In the pursuit of well-being, it's vital to pause and celebrate the milestones you achieve along the way. Whether you've embarked on a fitness journey, embraced a healthier lifestyle, or cultivated mindfulness through practices like chair yoga, every step forward is a reason for celebration. Recognize that well-being is not just a destination but a continuous journey, and each moment of progress deserves acknowledgment.

Take time to reflect on how far you've come. Celebrate the physical strength you've gained, the stress you've managed, and the inner peace you've found. These achievements are not just checkboxes but milestones in your lifelong pursuit of well-being.

Share your successes with loved ones, friends, or a supportive community. Your journey can inspire and uplift others on their paths to well-being. Through celebration and sharing, you foster a sense of connection and encouragement that amplifies the positive impact of your progress.

Remember that self-care and self-compassion are essential components of well-being. Celebrate not only your external achievements but also the inner growth, resilience, and self-awareness you've cultivated. Treat yourself with kindness and acknowledge that progress, no matter how small, is a testament to your dedication and determination.

As you celebrate your progress and well-being, stay open to continued growth and exploration. Embrace new challenges and opportunities that come your way, and let them enrich your journey. The pursuit of well-being is a dynamic and ever-evolving endeavor, and each step you take contributes to a healthier, happier, and more fulfilled life. So, celebrate your well-being journey, for it is a celebration of life itself.

Your feedback is incredibly valuable to me. Please take a moment to leave a review, sharing your thoughts and insights. Your input will help me refine future editions and continue assisting others on their path to rejuvenation.

Thank you for choosing this book as your companion. May your golden years continue to shine with newfound vitality and joy.

Printed in Great Britain
by Amazon

37376311R00066